WOMEN
AND
HEART DISEASE

An Epidemic

WOMEN
AND
HEART
DISEASE

An Epidemic

Lawrence J. Santora, MD
Shalizeh Shokooh, MD
Kelly Tucker, MD

Acknowledgements

Medicine is part science and part art. The science part requires years of study, constant review and assimilation of the latest scientific studies. The art part is more difficult. It is the art of medicine that makes great doctors. The art develops after interacting with thousands of patients over many years. The art develops from making decisions based on the fine subtleties of a physical exam, or on the nuances of a patient's words during an interview. It is the development of this art that may lead to a diagnosis that no textbook could readily provide. The practice of cardiology, despite the abundance of high technology, still relies on the art of the history and physical.

We dedicate this book to our patients who honor us with the privilege of providing their medical care. Our patients teach us our art. We hope through this book we may once again teach them. Perhaps one paragraph, one sentence, or even one word may bring home a truth leading to a treatment that may save a life.

We also dedicate this book to our families, whose patience, understanding and support allow us to practice our art. We would like to acknowledge the immense help of Donald Gazzaniga, Suzanne Byerley, Jennifer Tucker, MD, and Friedrich Roessler, MD in bringing this book to fruition. Finally, Rina Santora, RN, deserves special recognition for her many hours spent reviewing the manuscript and helping with the layout of this book.

Lawrence Santora, MD
Shalizeh Shokooh, MD
Kelly Tucker, MD

OC HEART HEALTH BOOKS
United States Copyright 2008 by Lawrence J. Santora, MD
WOMEN AND HEART DISEASE
New Revised Edition

This book is not intended to serve as a substitute for a physician. Nor is the authors' intent to give medical advice contrary to that of an attending physician.

Cover Painting by Lawrence Santora, MD
Painting is a rendition of Claude Monet's *Woman With The Umbrella.*
The woman's red dress is the American Heart Association's symbol for women and heart disease.

www.ocheart.org
www.arrowhead-classics.com

ISBN 1-886571-25-2
EAN 978-1-886571-25-9

10 9 8 7 6 5 4 3

Contents

Even though women under 50 get fewer heart attacks than men of the same age, they are twice as likely to die.

Introduction

More women die from heart disease than the next seven causes of death combined. Cardiovascular disease became the number one killer in women in 1908, only eight years after it became the number one killer for men. A century later, the trend of cardiovascular disease in women has not changed. Only through education can this trend be reversed. Only through knowledge can the epidemic be stopped. It is time for women to take control of their health, to find out what heart disease is, what puts one at risk, and how to prevent and treat heart disease appropriately.

According to the findings published in the *New England Journal of Medicine,* women are more likely than men to die of heart attacks. Since 1984, despite the advances in medical technology and knowledge, more young women have been dying from cardiovascular disease than men.

Men under 50 have more heart attacks than women in this age group, but more women than men die from their first heart attack. These are disturbing findings. It becomes more disturbing when we know that one out of two women will have some kind of heart disease and one in three will die from it. That counts for about half a million women dying from cardiovascular disease per year in this country.

The disparity in women and men can be attributed to many factors, some well known, and some not yet well understood. But, more and more we are finding that gender differences do exist and that women are not treated as aggressively as men when it comes to their hearts.

Jody's is one story we hope to hear less and less often as better knowledge leads to better treatment of women with heart disease. Jody was rushed to an emergency room at a large Seattle hospital after she complained of shoulder and neck pain. The doctor on duty examined her and asked her about her life and daily work habits. She mentioned that she was the mother of four children under ten years of age. He diagnosed the problem as stress. She was given a prescription for a medication to relieve the symptoms of stress and was sent home with her husband. Eighteen hours later, while her husband and two sons were at a ballgame, she died of a massive heart attack.

Many times emergency rooms are caught off guard when a woman under the age of 50 is brought in for evaluation of possible heart related symptoms. Emergency medical staffs often overlook a possible heart attack in these women due to their outward appearance of youth and good health. Symptoms of upper back pain, breathlessness, dizziness, and nausea are often attributed to non cardiac causes. One of the rules of emergency departments is to allow those with chest pain (possibly a heart attack) to go into emergency care ahead of all other patients. However, since many of the symptoms of heart attack in younger women are not the typical chest pain felt by the older male heart attack patient, these women are not readily identified. The younger woman suffering from a heart attack then may wait an hour or longer for attention. Many women may not receive life-saving treatments, such as artery-opening therapies, in a timely enough fashion.

Surveys have shown that only one out of three primary care doctors talk to their female patients about their hearts. And since women are less likely to perceive heart disease as their most important health concern, they are less likely to ask about their risks or to bring up their symptoms. Fortunately, awareness of heart disease in women is growing and hospitals and cardiac centers are dedicating more time and effort to addressing the problem.

Throughout the book, we will give detailed explanations of

symptoms, state of the art testing, medications and treatments. For example, simple ECG (electrocardiogram) stress tests are often a much less reliable indicator of heart disease in women than in men.

In the United States, women make up 52 % of the population, are expected to live longer than men, and be the care-givers in their families. Both doctors and patients need to be more proactive to prevent, diagnose, and treat the disease that claims so many lives each day. The knowledge you gain from this book may one day save your life.

1

What Is Heart Disease and How to Detect It

Heart disease refers to the damage or malfunction of any of the components of the heart. Since the heart is basically a pump, any malfunction can result in ineffective pumping action leading to symptoms or possibly death. A brief explanation of each of the heart's components makes it easier to understand the symptoms that may result from malfunction and what type of testing may be needed to detect the problem.

The coronary arteries

When most people think of heart disease, they think of a heart attack. Heart attacks are caused by plaque build up in the coronary arteries, and coronary artery disease is by far the most common type of heart disease.

The heart muscle

The heart is a pump about the size of your fist, consisting of muscular walls that do the pumping of blood.

The heart valves

There are four heart valves—small, fibrous tissue that like tiny doors allow the blood to flow in one direction through the heart chambers. They are vital to consistent flow that in turn moves the blood along without flooding the heart chambers.

The electrical conduction system

Nerve fibers embedded in the heart muscle to feed and control its electrical activity and rhythm are referred to as the conduction system.

The pericardium

A fibrous sac called the pericardium surrounds the outside of the heart.

1. Coronary Artery Disease

A heart attack refers to actual damage to the heart muscle. Some heart attacks are small, meaning there is very little damage to the pumping function of the heart, and some may be so severe they lead to such a large degree of pump damage that congestive heart failure results. When congestive heart failure develops, shortness of breath and an inability to exercise occurs. A significant decrease in the overall quality of life can result. Half of all heart attacks result in sudden death. This means that when the coronary artery suddenly closes, the heart muscle is deprived of blood leading to a deadly heart rhythm called ventricular fibrillation. Unless cardiopulmonary resuscitation is started and the heart is defibrillated (electrically shocked back into normal rhythm) death occurs in minutes.

So as a result of coronary artery disease, we have at one end of the spectrum, catastrophic sudden death or severe congestive heart failure, and at the other end we may have ongoing chest discomfort due to a constricted coronary artery. This chest discomfort (referred to as angina pectoris) can be very mild or quite disabling, and can be treated in a number of ways, from medicine to coronary bypass surgery, described in detail in subsequent chapters.

Atherosclerosis or hardening of the coronary arteries is the major cause of heart attacks. Therefore, most testing and screening for heart disease involves tests to detect disease (plaque) in the coronary arteries.

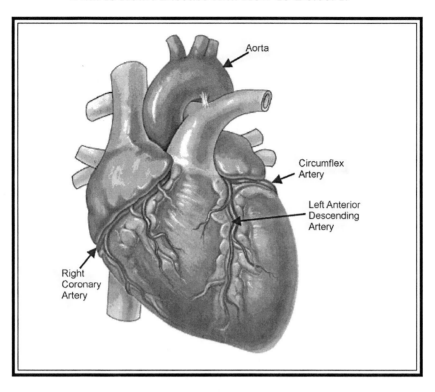

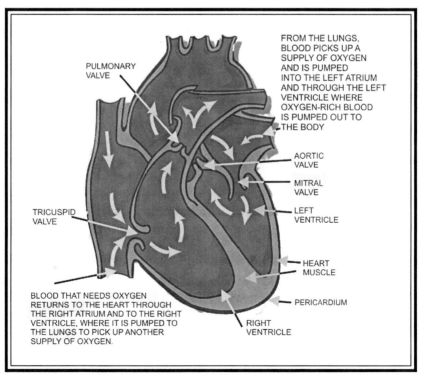

The Formation of Plaque in the Coronary

To understand the difficulty in detecting coronary heart disease, you need a brief understanding of how plaque develops in the coronary arteries. Plaque starts out slowly, usually as thin deposits of cholesterol and fat, referred to as *fatty streaks*, in the lining (called the endothelium) of the coronary artery wall. Tobacco smoke, high blood pressure, an infection that leads to inflammation, and numerous other factors can cause small fissures or cracks to form in the normally smooth lining of the endothelium. These fissures then allow the fatty deposits to adhere to the lining. Your body's response is to try to heal the irritated lining by having white blood cells engulf the fatty streaks. A soft plaque develops in the lining of the artery consisting of fatty substances, cholesterol, fibrous tissue, and white blood cells.

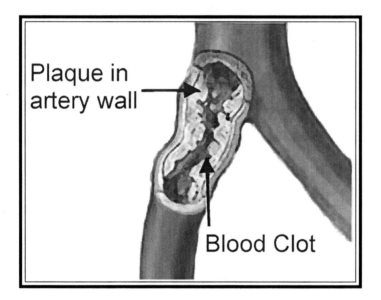

Plaque in artery wall

Blood Clot

As time goes on, the plaque enlarges and calcium deposits in the soft plaque form a hard calcified plaque, hence the term atherosclerosis or hardening of the arteries. Eventually, the opening of the artery starts to narrow. With time, unless risk factors are modified (lowering cholesterol, stopping smoking, etc.) the plaque can gradually enlarge leading to a reduction of blood flow causing angina or chest discomfort.

A second common scenario is that at some critical point, the plaque suddenly develops a fissure on its surface and ruptures. This sudden rupturing of the plaque causes a clot to form on its surface which completely blocks blood flow in the coronary artery and causes a heart attack.

The gradual narrowing may need to be treated with medications, angioploasty, stents or bypass surgery (see Chapter 5). A stress test will detect plaque if the artery is narrowed about 70% or more. If the artery has significant plaque, but no segment of plaque is narrowing the artery by at least 70%, the stress test can be normal.

The frightening part of the plaque formation process is that *most heart attacks occur when a minor plaque that is not restricting blood flow, suddenly ruptures and is therefore not detected beforehand by a stress test.* Most people have a friend or relative that was thought to be perfectly healthy, no symptoms and then, suddenly dies of a heart attack. That person had plaque that was not restricting blood flow, therefore, no warning signs or symptoms, until the plaque suddenly ruptured. A stress test could very well have been normal if performed a few days before these episodes of sudden death.

Detecting Coronary Artery Disease: Non-invasive techniques

So how do we detect plaque that is silent until it suddenly ruptures and causes a heart attack or death? Fortunately, we now have amazing technology that allows us to simply and non-invasively detect this plaque. Electron Beam Computed Tomography (EBCT) scans pick up the presence of this "silent" plaque in the coronary artery. They are the most accurate non-invasive method to detect plaque and determine the risk for a heart attack.

Fast Fact
EBCT heart scans are recommended by the American Heart Association for people of intermediate risk of heart disease

---

A. Electron Beam CT heart scans (EBCT)

EBCT scans are the most sensitive and accurate noninvasive test to pick up the presence of plaque in the coronary arteries in the asymptomatic person. The EBCT scanner is a very fast version of the traditional CT scan. Because of its speed, it can take clear and accurate pictures of the calcium (calcium is part of the plaque) in the coronary arteries and is the only CT scan approved by the FDA for coronary calcium screening. The scanner measures calcium in the coronary arteries three dimensionally and then calculates a total calcium score. The higher the calcium score, the more plaque.

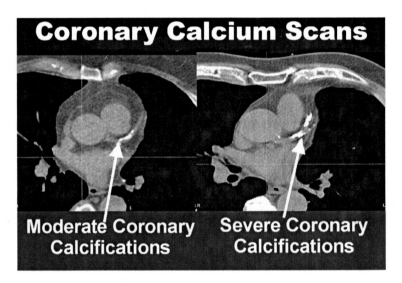

Coronary Calcium Scans

Moderate Coronary Calcifications   **Severe Coronary Calcifications**

A calcium percentile also compares your score to other women your age. If for instance, you are forty years old and have a calcium score of 70, you have a calcium percentile of 90%. This does not mean you have a 90% chance of a heart attack, it simply means that you have more plaque than 90% of the women your age. It means that your plaque needs aggressive treatment. Incidentally, calcium in the plaque formation has nothing to do with the calcium you eat or that you may be taking to prevent osteoporosis. You can take in all the calcium you want without increasing your risk of plaque formation in your coronary arteries.

The higher the calcium score and the higher the percentile,

the more likely the future chance of a heart attack or the need for invasive procedures *unless* you modify your risk factors. The total calcium score is more predictive of a future cardiac event than all other traditional risk factors. So, who should have an EBCT scan?

Indications for EBCT heart scans:

Fast Fact

Do not rely on cholesterol ratios! Go by the absolute number of total cholesterol, HDL and LDL cholesterol

---

Any woman over 40 with at least one of these risk factors:
- High blood pressure
- High cholesterol (even if the HDL is high)
- Family history of heart disease
- Smoking
- Diabetes
- Metabolic syndrome
- Low HDL (low level of the good cholesterol)
- Obesity

Note: If you are having symptoms, for instance, chest discomfort or shortness of breath, you should contact your physician first, before getting an EBCT heart scan.

The EBCT scan reports the total calcium score, the calcium percentile, and a calcium volume. Based on the above three numbers, the cardiologist may recommend the following:

- New target level of total cholesterol, LDL, HDL and triglycerides. The higher your calcium score and calcium percentile, the lower you should get your cholesterol levels.
- Need for further tests, such as a stress echocardiogram and advanced lipid testing. The higher the calcium score, the higher the chance that plaque is restricting blood flow. Since stress tests detect severe restriction in blood flow, you may need a stress test if the calcium score is high.

Future surveillance of calcium score. When should the EBCT scan be repeated? If there is no calcium, in general a repeat scan is not needed for four to five years. If calcium is present, then a repeat scan is usually needed in 18 to 24 months to determine if the therapy is working. You may have started therapy with a goal of getting your LDL cholesterol down to 100. How do you know it's working? You don't know unless you start to get symptoms of chest pain or repeat the EBCT. In general, if the calcium volume does not increase by more than 10% per year, you are getting effective treatment and are in a safe zone of control.

The following histories offer common examples in which the EBCT scan was invaluable in helping to make treatment decisions.

Marge — Does her low HDL cholesterol need to be treated?
Marge was a 50-year-old medical doctor. She was of normal weight, exercised four to five times a week since college. No symptoms and no other risk factors. It was difficult to convince her, fit and healthy looking as she claimed to be, to take a medicine to raise the HDL.

She was well aware that the HDL cholesterol protects the heart and if the HDL is low, there is a risk of coronary disease. Her EBCT revealed a very high calcium score of 300, placing her in the 90th percentile at high risk of future heart attack.

Marge started on niacin, one of the few effective medications to raise HDL. The HDL went from 30 to 70 and a repeat EBT scan two years later showed a reduction in plaque. The calcium score decreased to 280! It is our belief that the scan saved her life. Why? If she had had no treatment she would not have known she had coronary artery disease until she had a heart attack.

Keep in mind that untreated plaque in your heart can progress up to 30% or more per year. With proper treatment, the plaque can be stabilized and progression slowed or reversed. The time to treat plaque is before you have symptoms or a heart attack.

Donna — Does she need cholesterol treatment?

Donna had mildly high cholesterol and no family history of heart disease. Her physical exam was unremarkable other than her being perhaps 20 pounds overweight. At 58 years old, a former professional athlete, she continued a vigorous exercise program. She showed no symptoms and no other risk factors for heart disease. In fact, she was the youngest of nine siblings, none of whom had heart disease. She came for a routine cardiac evaluation.

Total cholesterol was only slightly high at 218, the HDL, LDL, and triglycerides were reasonable. A stress echocardiogram registered borderline abnormal. Should the cholesterol be treated with medications? It was only borderline high. Didn't lack of heart disease in the family count? Didn't the fact that she had no symptoms count? Perhaps. Nevertheless, she agreed to an EBCT heart scan.

The score was extremely high, greater than 3000! Next Donna had an invasive angiogram which revealed two of the three coronary arteries were totally blocked. She went on to have four-vessel coronary bypass surgery. There is no question that had she not checked in she would have had a heart attack. Two years later she's doing great on a combination of niacin and a statin and her cholesterol profile is perfect. There is no question the scan saved her life.

Susan — High total cholesterol but high HDL cholesterol—is she protected?

High cholesterol, but high HDL cholesterol was the case with Susan, a 48-year-old former marathon runner, still in excellent shape, no symptoms and no other risk factors. Susan's total cholesterol had hovered around 240 for years, however the HDL was quite high at around 90 to 100. This is a common picture in women. Their cholesterol has not been treated because it has been thought that the high HDL is "protective," somehow imposing immunity from heart disease. Susan's total cholesterol to HDL ratio of 2.4 was very good. Don't be fooled by ratios!

A stress test, as expected, was normal and not helpful in answering the question of whether she should have her cholesterol treated. An EBCT scan showed a high calcium score. It was clear that Susan had developed coronary disease from high total cholesterol. The high HDL cholesterol was not protective in her case. She is now on a statin and her total cholesterol is normal. She will have her EBCT scan repeated in two years to see if the treatment is effective in slowing the progression of plaque.

Janis — Is her treatment effective?

Janis was a 51-year-old with high blood pressure and high cholesterol. We had treated her for 15 years with medications and maintained perfect blood pressure and cholesterol control. No symptoms and no other risk factors. She heard about the EBCT scan and we thought it would give a good baseline of her status.

We fully expected the scan to be normal or perhaps only slightly abnormal. After all, she did see us every six months for fifteen years, had excellent control of her risk factors and had several stress echocardiograms through the years, all normal. To our shock, her EBCT calcium score was over 400. Was this a failure of therapy? An advanced lipid panel measured the size of the LDL particle and the subcomponents of the HDL particles. (These tests are explained in more detail in the following chapters.) These results revealed her LDL cholesterol was unusually small in size, which is more likely to cause plaque. Also, the HDL 2b component, which is the portion that actually scavenges the plaque out of the artery, was unusually low. Niacin was added to her statin regimen to correct these two problems.

Did we do her any good for the past fifteen years? We think we did. If her cholesterol had not been treated, we are convinced she would have had a heart attack years ago. She was treated with the state-of-the-art approach as we knew it in the late 1980's and 1990's. State-of-the-art nowadays, we believe, is the EBCT scan. As important, the EBCT scan also tells us who does not need treatment. For instance, if your cholesterol is high and your EBCT scan does not show calcium, then you probably can avoid medications and be treated with diet and exercise.

In summary: EBCT heart scans are absolutely the most accurate non-invasive method to detect coronary heart disease. The scan tells if you do or do not have disease. If you have disease, it can be quantified, your risk of a heart attack determined and proper treatment rendered to prevent a heart attack. Just as important, it tells you if you do not need treatment. Not everyone with high cholesterol or low HDL needs treatment with medications.

Approaching heart disease using EBCT heart scans for coronary calcium screening not only makes good medical sense, but also good financial sense. Not everyone with cardiac risk factors develops coronary disease. An EBCT heart scan costs less than $400. If the scan does not show calcium, you can potentially avoid the $1,500 per year cost for cholesterol medications, associated lab tests costs, and potential side effects from the medications. There are additional benefits. Other structures in the chest are scanned at the same time. It is not uncommon to pick up tumors of the lung (especially in smokers) when the tumors are so small they are not detected on chest x-rays. This early detection leads to a much higher chance of cure. Also, aneurysms of the aorta, calcified plaque in the aorta that may lead to strokes, enlarged lymph nodes and numerous other abnormalities are frequently detected with the EBCT scan. Unlike other types of CT scans, the EBCT heart scan is extremely accurate and fast and delivers very low radiation exposure. The radiation dose is often one-fifth to one-tenth of a conventional CT scan.

B. CT Angiography of the coronary arteries

Fast Fact
CT angiography is not a screening test! It is used if you have symptoms or an abnormal stress test.

CT angiography of the coronary arteries is the newest **non-invasive** way to actually visualize the coronary arteries using the EBCT scan or 64 slice CT scan. An angiogram means taking pictures of an artery. Traditionally, the only way to actually take pictures or angiograms of the coronary arteries is to perform a heart catheterization and invasive coronary angiogram. In this procedure, we thread a small tube or catheter into the artery in the leg, then we place the catheter directly into the coronary artery, inject dye and take pictures of the dye flowing into the arteries. This reveals the degree of obstruction or narrowing by plaque in the coronary artery.

The CT angiogram is non-invasive. We do not enter the arteries with a catheter and no hospitalization or special preparation is needed. We inject a small quantity of standard X-ray dye into a vein in the arm. You hold your breath for 30 seconds and the scan will reproduce an angiogram of the coronary arteries almost as precise as an invasive coronary angiogram. There is little risk (unless an allergy to iodine or X-ray contrast dyes or kidney malfunction are present).

The following are indications for a CT angiogram based on the recommendations of your physician:

• Patients who have had prior coronary bypass surgery and have had a change in symptoms or a stress test that is not conclusive. Remember that the coronary bypass grafts tend to close over time and it is best to detect impending graft closure before a heart attack occurs.
• Patients who have not had surgery but have chest pain and their stress test is not conclusive.
• Patients who have not had surgery but have weakened heart muscle, also called a cardiomyopathy, to see if coronary artery blockages are the cause.

The following is an example of a patient who benefited from the CT angiogram.

Lilly – Are her coronary bypass grafts functioning?
An 82 year-old woman who had coronary bypass surgery 12 years earlier. We knew that by ten years post surgery up to 70% of the bypass grafts are closed or are about to close. Lilly started to have angina (chest pain) for the first time since surgery.

She underwent a simple 15 minute CT angiogram that revealed all the grafts were open except the one to the artery in the back of the heart (the circumflex artery). We know that not all the coronary arteries are of equal importance. It depends on how much heart muscle is supplied by that artery.

In general, the arteries in the back of the heart are the least vital and problems with the grafts to those arteries can often be treated with medications, as opposed to a stent or repeat open-heart surgery. Keep in mind that Lilly was 82. We decided it was safe to treat her without doing an invasive coronary angiogram, which although relatively safe, requires a hospital admission time of at least six to ten hours, and costs $10,000 to $15,000. We decided on a $1,500 CT angiogram using the same EBCT heart scanner plus the injection of dye into the arm vein. This offered us the same answers, at no risk, no incision. What is more amazing, Lilly drove herself to the test and went out to lunch afterwards.

C. Resting ECG

The ECG (electrocardiogram), though somewhat useful in a patient with symptoms of chest pain or palpitations, is of little help in screening the general female population to determine heart disease. It is a quick and inexpensive test but even if the ECG is normal, it provides very little reassurance that heart disease is not present. In fact, it is most helpful only if it is abnormal. At least half the people who arrive at emergency with a heart attack will have a normal ECG.

To detect obstruction of blood flow to the heart, the heart needs to be stressed with exercise or drugs. These tests are described in more detail in the following sections.

D. Stress Testing

Fast Fact
A stress test will only become abnormal if an artery is narrowed more than 70%

As mentioned earlier, stress tests detect plaque that restricts blood flow, which means that it picks up advanced heart disease that likely needs to be corrected with open heart surgery or stents. Each type of stress test has different degrees of accuracy and limitations. Similarly, the time involved, the complexity of performance and cost for each test is different and therefore, the proper test should be determined by a physician.

We use stress testing as an indirect measurement of blood flow in the coronary arteries. A coronary artery usually narrows around 60 to 70% before blood flow is restricted enough to cause a reduction of flow during exercise. An artery can be severely narrowed, yet an ECG taken at rest can be normal because the heart needs less blood flow at rest. On the other hand, during exercise the blood flow needs of the heart are increased and the ECG during stress will often become abnormal if the artery is significantly narrowed.

If a stress test is normal, it doesn't mean the coronary arteries are normal. There may be narrowing in the arteries and plaque that is not yet restricting flow, but could at some time cause a heart attack should the plaque suddenly rupture.

We get the best information about non-flow limiting plaque with the EBCT heart scan. Although a stress test is usually done to help diagnose the presence of obstructive coronary artery disease, sometimes it is done to evaluate exercise capacity in a patient with valvular or congenital heart disease.

At times, a stress test is done in patients who suffer from cardiac arrhythmias to try to induce or reproduce those abnormal heart rhythms. Here are the basics about the various types of stress tests:

Simple Treadmill Stress Testing

An exercise stress test is also called a stress electrocardiogram. It records your heartbeat while you walk on a treadmill or ride on a stationary bike. This test helps your doctor evaluate the cause of chest pain. It also measures the exercise capacity of your heart after a heart attack or surgery.

The patient has to walk uphill on a treadmill, and sometimes jog, to achieve his or her maximum heart rate. The ECG is observed and recorded throughout the exercise and for about five minutes in the recovery stage after exercise. Changes in the ECG are observed as the heart rate increases (that is, as the heart is stressed) and compared to the ECG at rest, before exercise. A special section of the ECG, called the ST segment, is measured as an indicator of "ischemia" which means inadequate blood flow to the heart.

When positive, or abnormal, ECG changes occur with typical chest pain. When chest pain and ECG changes occur together during the exercise test, then the simple treadmill test is very useful. Unfortunately, without nuclear or echocardiographic imaging, a simple treadmill test will often give falsely positive or falsely negative results, therefore, they are not very accurate at predicting disease by themselves.

Patients with heart disease can have a normal treadmill (false negative test), and sometimes people with normal hearts can have an abnormal treadmill (false positive test). To improve the accuracy of stress testing to detect advanced heart disease, more advanced and complex stress tests are used. A simple treadmill stress test is the least expensive and least accurate of all stress tests, especially in women. A stress echocardiogram or nuclear stress test should be used to determine if coronary artery blockages are present in women.

Nuclear Stress Testing

Often your treadmill test will include nuclear imaging. Cardiolite and Thallium are the two types of nuclear material, also referred to as the nuclear tracer, that is injected to make the pictures.

Cardiac nuclear imaging is sometimes called a perfusion scan. Performing a stress test with the addition of Thallium or Cardiolite imaging greatly enhances accuracy since they are selectively taken up from the blood by heart muscle. The present protocols use a combined approach employing both agents.

The tracer, made up of a small amount of radioactive matter, is given to you through a vein in your arm. A camera scans the tracer in the blood as it flows through your heart muscle. We do this scan before, during, and after exercise and then compare blood flow at rest and during exercise to see differences.

You lie comfortably on a table under a nuclear camera while the scanner is taking the heart image. When the picture is complete, you exercise on a treadmill or stationary bike until you approach a certain predetermined heart rate with age taken into consideration. This is the target heart rate. The Cardiolite is then injected into an arm vein and you exercise for about a minute more to circulate the tracer through the heart.

You then lie under the same imaging camera for about 15 to 20 minutes to gain the "stress images." The rest and exercise pictures are then compared to determine if there is a blocked artery. If all the coronary arteries are open, then the radioactive tracer will fill the surface of the heart muscle in a uniform manner. Your heart will appear somewhat like a donut or a pie. If a coronary artery is blocked, the area of the heart muscle supplied by the blocked artery will not get the radioactive tracer and the image will look like a "bite" taken out of a donut or a slice taken out of a pie.

Your doctor will then have an indicator that is about 90% accurate. It will reveal a significantly narrowed artery if there is a problem. Depending on your age, related symptoms, and the size of the defect on the scan, your physician may decide that an invasive angiogram is needed, or perhaps a CT angiogram.

Although nuclear stress tests are very accurate, they are not cheap. The radioisotope itself costs several hundred dollars. The equipment used to image the heart costs hundreds of thousands of dollars, and expert nuclear technicians with computer skills are required. Such nuclear stress tests may cost between $1,200 and $1,800.

Stress Echocardiogram

This is an exercise stress test using ultrasound images of your heart muscle to improve the diagnostic accuracy of stress testing. Your heart muscle wall motion is evaluated at rest, and then again at peak exercise using ultrasound images. If there is a blocked artery (coronary artery disease) causing your chest pain, then the echocardiogram images will show weakness in the muscle fed by the blocked artery at peak exercise. Normally, the heart muscle wall contracts and moves more vigorously immediately after exercise than when the heart is at rest.

The finding of decreased wall motion after exercise is a reliable indicator that the heart is not getting enough blood through the coronary arteries to meet the needs of the exercising heart. Therefore, a wall motion abnormality is a sign of narrowed coronary artery. The echocardiogram has some advantage over the nuclear stress test in that the stress echocardiogram gives detailed images of the heart valves, the thickness of the heart muscle walls as well as the sack around the heart (pericardium).

The stress echocardiogram also requires less time to perform. However, since the echocardiogram is an ultrasound test, in some patients the images are not optimal due to the interference of the overlying lung tissue, breast tissues, and excess body fat. Furthermore, certain abnormal heart rhythms and certain ECG abnormalities make interpreting wall motion more difficult. Because of these limitations, a nuclear stress test may be a better test in certain circumstances. For women, a nuclear or stress echocardiogram should be used, not just a simple treadmill stress test, if one wants to determine if a coronary artery is restricted. In addition, both the nuclear and the echocardiogram stress test also give information about the pumping function of the heart. This pumping function is referred to as the left ventricular *ejection fraction,* described in more detail below.

What If You Can't Exercise?

Some patients can't exercise because of disabilities such as arthritis, recent injuries, surgery, or obesity. In these cases we can use pharmacologic stimulation to simulate exercise. With nuclear stress tests we use intravenous (IV) adenosine or dipyridamole (IV Dipy) to stimulate the heart. With stress echocardiograms we usually use Dobutamine. These medicines may precipitate chest pain, but their effects can be quickly reversed with medications.

Before Your Stress Test

When you schedule your stress test, be sure to mention the medicines you're taking and ask if you should take any before the test. This will vary according to your medications. Don't eat, smoke, or drink alcohol for four hours before the test. Caffeine may interfere with certain types of nuclear stress tests, so ask if caffeine is permissible the day of your test. Make sure to wear a two piece outfit. This allows for placement of the ECG monitoring leads on your chest. You may need to undress from the waist up and put on a short hospital gown. You also need to wear good walking shoes.

E. Other Tests for Heart Structure and Function

Fast Fact
The ejection fraction is the most important measurement of heart function

---

The *ejection fraction (EF)* is the most important number you should know. It is one of the most important determinations of heart function and is the most important factor in predicting a patient's risk of dying suddenly from a cardiac arrhythmia or congestive heart failure. The ejection fraction measures the pumping function of the heart. The heart at rest fills the left ventricle, the main pumping chamber, with oxygen rich blood draining from the lungs. Then, the left ventricle chamber contracts and ejects the blood into the aorta and directs the blood to the rest of the body. If 60% of the blood is ejected from the left ventricle chamber, then the ejection fraction is 60%. An ejection fraction greater than 50% is normal. An ejection fraction below 35 to 40% is severely abnormal.

The ejection fraction is a rough measure of a heart muscle's strength and determines how much damage has occurred. An EF can also be calculated by an echocardiogram or part of the nuclear stress testing scans or MUGA scans (which use a radioisotope injected into an arm vein). An ejection fraction is also measured during a left ventriculogram done at the time of cardiac catheterization or a non-invasive CT angiogram using the EBCT heart scan.

Some patients, especially those who have lung disease or who are obese, fail to obtain an adequate echocardiogram due to the ultrasound's inability to image the heart. In such cases, nuclear scans are the best option to determine an ejection fraction.

Myocardial Viability Scans

Myocardial viability scans are used to see if a weakened heart muscle still has the potential for recovery or is permanently damaged. They are used only under certain circumstances when determining if the heart muscle is viable (still a living heart muscle, i.e., not a scar tissue) to determine if efforts to improve blood flow via bypass surgery or angioplasty might recover contractile heart muscle strength if blood flow is restored. If the heart muscle is dead, then new blood flow will be of no benefit and the risk of surgery or angioplasty can be avoided. The PET scan (Positron Emission Tomography) is a type of resting nuclear scan that is the most accurate but less readily available test to determine viability. Thallium double injection two day scans are another method used to determine viability.

Resting Echocardiography

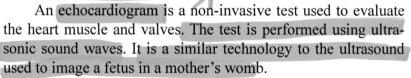

An echocardiogram is a non-invasive test used to evaluate the heart muscle and valves. The test is performed using ultrasonic sound waves. It is a similar technology to the ultrasound used to image a fetus in a mother's womb.

Echocardiograms are a quick and cost effective test for accurately defining the heart muscle strength and function, the size of the cardiac chambers, and the function of the heart valves. In addition, it is an excellent way to determine the presence or absence of a pericardial effusion (water around the heart in the pericardial sac).

We perform an echocardiogram by placing a transducer that produces sound waves on the chest wall. A gel is placed on the skin under the transducer to enhance sound wave transmission. The images received from the reflected sound waves are then recorded digitally or on a video tape. The test generally takes about thirty minutes and causes no side effects. Sometimes an adequate quality echocardiogram cannot be obtained. Sound waves penetrate tissue and water well, but do not penetrate bone or air without distortion. The quality of the echo image is reduced if the patient has emphysema or asthma, which causes the hyper-expanded lungs to interfere with the transducer's ability to obtain a clear picture.

Common cardiac disorders evaluated by the echocardiogram:
- *Cardiomyopathy*

This is a condition in which the heart muscle becomes weak and can result in congestive heart failure.

- *Heart Valve Disease*

Mitral valve prolapse, aortic valve or mitral valve stenosis (narrowing), or regurgitation (leakage) are forms of heart valve disease. Endocarditis, which is an infection of the heart valve, is also best determined with echocardiography.

- *Coronary artery disease*

Prior heart attacks or scar tissue can be identified by viewing the wall motion injury that resulted.

- *Pericardial Disease*

Fluid or scarring and thickening of the sack around the heart can be identified.

Transesophageal Echocardiogram (TEE)

Sometimes, due to a patient's body configuration, a good echo cannot be obtained from the chest wall. In these cases, we can get excellent images by performing a TEE.

A TEE is a transesophageal echocardiogram. This procedure is performed when improved images are required, or when there is a specific concern about the left atrium or mitral valve. The esophagus sits right next to the rear of the heart without lung or bone to interfere with echo imaging.

A TEE is performed using sedation to suppress the gag reflex in the back of the throat. A lubricated transducer is then gently slipped down the throat to the middle of the esophagus. With the patient sedated, the images are obtained. The test takes about twenty minutes to perform and usually requires about one hour for the sedation to resolve.

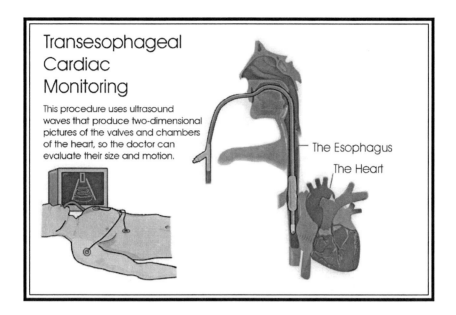

Transesophageal Cardiac Monitoring

This procedure uses ultrasound waves that produce two-dimensional pictures of the valves and chambers of the heart, so the doctor can evaluate their size and motion.

The Esophagus

The Heart

Invasive Testing For Heart Disease

Cardiac Catheterization and Coronary Angiogram

A cardiac catheterization or cardiac cath refers to a procedure done to evaluate the heart using catheters, pre-shaped, hollow tubes that can be slid up a vein or artery to the heart. Through these catheters pressure can be measured, oxygen saturation determined, or contrast dye injected.

Most are performed to determine if there are blocked coronary arteries. The angiogram is used to further determine what causes a stress test to be abnormal or to further investigate the cause of chest pain. Other indications to perform a coronary angiogram are to determine the cause of congestive heart failure, or abnormalities of the heart valves, such as the severity of narrowing (stenosis) of the valves or the amount of leakage (regurgitation). A heart catheterization is almost always done before coronary bypass surgery can be performed and certainly prior to PTCA or stents (discussed in Chapter 5).

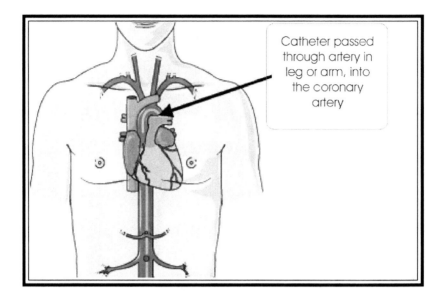

Catheter passed through artery in leg or arm, into the coronary artery

Invasive Cardiac Cath and Coronary Angiogram Procedure

The patient is mildly sedated and a site is chosen to enter the vein and artery. The site can be in the arm, through an artery in the wrist (radial artery) or near the elbow (brachial artery); but most commonly it is done via the femoral artery in the groin. The site is sterilized and local anesthesia is achieved using a subcutaneous injection of Lidocaine. There is no discomfort once the skin is numbed. A hollow needle is used to puncture the artery. Through the needle a flexible wire (guide wire) is passed into the artery. Once this guide wire is inserted, the needle is withdrawn and a sheath is threaded over the wire into the artery. The guide wire is then withdrawn.

The sheath is a flexible tube with a one way exterior valve. This allows the cardiologist to pass catheters into the sheath and into the artery/vein, but prevents blood from exiting. Through the sheath a catheter is then passed up to the heart using X-ray fluoroscopy to guide the catheter.

The catheter is then positioned in various chambers to measure pressure and oxygen levels, and to inject contrast dye. Contrast dye can be used to take a picture of the contracting ventricle, providing visualization of the heart muscle's contractile strength. Contrast dye can also be injected into the coronary arteries, providing a picture of those arteries and revealing any atherosclerotic plaque (obstructive hardening of the arteries). This portion of the test is referred to as a coronary angiogram. If a PTCA or stent is the appropriate method to fix a blocked artery found at the time of the angiogram, the cardiologist will usually perform that procedure at the same time as the angiogram. If just an angiogram is performed, the patient is usually discharged the same day. If an intervention (PTCA or stent) is performed, the cardiologist will usually require the patient to stay in the hospital overnight. If open heart surgery is deemed to be the best treatment, the surgery is usually done the next day by a thoracic surgeon. (A cardiologist performs angiograms and interventions such as stents. Open-heart surgery is performed by a different type of physician who has a different training. They are referred to as cardiovascular/cardiothoracic surgeons.)

Post Catheterization Recovery

After the cardiac catheterization is completed, the catheters and sheaths are removed from the artery. Usually a closure device, a small plug, is inserted into the puncture site to seal the artery. Bed rest for one to two hours is needed. It is recommended that the patient avoid strenuous activity or deep knee bends for a day or two while the arterial puncture site heals completely.

Possible Complications of a Cardiac Catheterization

The most common complication is bleeding at the site of the arterial puncture. Usually, this is self limited and resolves with time. Sometimes this bleeding requires a transfusion. It rarely requires vascular surgery to repair the artery. Other complications include allergic reactions to the contrast dye, arrhythmia, stroke, and heart attack. These are very rare. In general, this is considered a safe exam that is done frequently and commonly.

Women have as much need as men — perhaps more so for women under 50 — to be alert to the variety of tests available for detection of heart disease.

2. Cardiomyopathy: *Heart Muscle Problems*

Damage to heart muscle is referred to as myocardial disease ("myo" means muscle, "cardial" means heart). So myocardial disease is a disease of the heart muscle, also called "cardiomyopathy." Damage to the heart muscle reduces the ability of the heart to pump adequate blood to meet the needs of the body. The consequence is usually shortness of breath with exercise, and if there is severe pump damage, fluid cannot be circulated adequately through the lungs, leading to shortness of breath at rest. When shortness of breath occurs at rest, the lungs are congested due to failure of the heart to pump, thus the term "congestive heart failure." The ejection fraction is the standard measurement of heart muscle function, which can be determined by echocardiograms, nuclear heart scans or angiogram of the left ventricle. Congestive heart failure and the latest treatments are discussed in the following chapters.

3. Heart Valve Disease

Damage to the heart valves is called *valvular heart disease*. The valves can be damaged from infection, congenital abnormalities, wear and tear with the aging process, or weakened if the surrounding heart muscle is damaged. The two valves on the left side of the heart, the mitral and the aortic, are much more commonly damaged than the right sided valves, the tricuspid and the pulmonic. The valves may be damaged in such a way that they leak blood backward (referred to as "regurgitation") or they can be narrowed (referred to as "stenosis") inhibiting the forward flow of blood through the heart chambers. The major symptoms, when the damage is severe, is shortness of breath, then less often chest pain, and less likely, fainting (see subsequent chapters.) Echocardiograms are the usual method of diagnosing heart valve problems. Heart catheterizations are used for more advanced disease to help determine if surgery is needed to repair the valves.

4. Malfunctioning of The Electrical Conduction System

Malfunction of the nerve fibers embedded in the heart muscle to feed and control its electrical activity and rhythm leads to arrhythmias or abnormalities of the heartbeat. Most of the abnormalities are harmless "premature beats" that are usually felt as skipped beats or palpitations. More serious rhythm problems can lead to loss of consciousness or even death. The usual initial evaluation is with a 24-hour Holter monitor. More advanced testing may require electrophysiological testing. Chapters on abnormal heart rhythms discuss this subject in detail.

5. Pericardial Disease

The pericardium is similar to the sac or covering around the lungs called the pleura. Most people are familiar with the term "pleurisy" which is an inflammation of the pleura often the result of an infection and often felt as a sharp pain with breathing. Damage to pericardium is called pericardial disease and is often due to an infection. However, the pericardium, when inflamed or infected can cause a build up of fluid between the sac and the surface of the heart (this space is called the pericardial space). The fluid can compress the heart and not only cause chest pain, but also severe shortness of breath. The echocardiogram is the most common tool to diagnose pericardial disease. The most common problem is called "pericarditis," or inflammation of the sac. This is usually treated with anti-inflammatory drugs such as ibuprofen and steroids such as prednisone. Usually pericarditis has a short and benign course.

2

Risk Factors and Heart Disease

KNOW YOUR NUMBERS

Michelle was a 35-year-old mother of one who came to our office because of her family history of heart disease. She was a smoker and overweight with a sedentary life style. She had been told her cholesterol was somewhat high, but did not know her levels. She had never thought about all her risk factors because she was young and no one had emphasized them to her. *Should she be concerned?*

Many factors can increase one's risk for heart disease. Hardening of the arteries of the heart and the rest of the body happen over a long period of time. Some risk factors are uncontrollable, but most of them can be modified by changing one's lifestyle. Cardiac risk factors have been shown through clinical and epidemiologic studies to increase risk for both women and men. The more risk factors involved, the higher the risk for having a heart attack. Fifty percent of patients with heart disease do not have conventional risk factors. However, in the case of women, 90% of those 45 and younger have at least one risk factor at the time of their presentation. They are more likely to be overweight, smoke, and lead a sedentary lifestyle.

What Cannot Be Controlled?

Age
We cannot control the fact that we all age, however, through a better and healthier lifestyle, we can prevent adding other risk factors to our portfolio. As women get older and pass menopause, they are at higher risk of dying from a heart attack than men.

Gender
Men are at higher risk of having heart disease and heart attacks especially early in life. Women tend to develop heart disease about 10 to 15 years later than men, probably due to the protective effect of estrogen before menopause.

Family History
According to scientific studies, the risk of heart disease increases if a parent or sibling had heart disease early in life. That means if the male relative was 55 years of age or younger and the female relative was 65 years of age or younger. A recent study showed a possibility of higher risk of heart disease when a sibling suffered from the disease. The sibling's heart disease probably reflects not only shared genetic susceptibility, but also shared lifestyle and dietary habits. Again, we cannot change the genes we inherit from our parents, but modification of the controllable risk factors does decrease our risk for heart disease and heart attack. Somehow, we develop a genetic tendency for our arteries to be more sensitive or more resistant to normal circulating cholesterol, or to the effects of tobacco smoke or blood pressure.

What Can We Control?

Hypertension (High Blood Pressure)
High blood pressure occurs when the systolic pressure (top number) is equal to or over 140 and the diastolic pressure (bottom number) is equal to or over 90 millimeters of mercury (mm Hg). High blood pressure does not have any specific symptoms;

therefore, there are many people who have high blood pressure for a long time before it is diagnosed. It affects many of the organs and structures in the body, including the heart, the kidneys, the brain, and the eyes. Since high blood pressure can damage vital organs long before symptoms develop, hypertension has been called a "silent killer."

Hypertension is more common after age 35, and for women, it becomes more prevalent as they pass menopause. In most people there is no specific cause for the increase in high blood pressure. In these cases, it is called essential hypertension. However, there are some secondary causes for hypertension stemming from the kidneys or from hormonal sources.

When we look at the most common risk factors for heart disease, hypertension is number one. It directly increases the risk for heart disease and eventually for a heart attack. When high blood pressure is combined with other risk factors, the risk of heart disease can increase several times.

For those predisposed to high blood pressure, certain medications and habits can contribute. Women who take birth control pills can be at a higher risk for developing hypertension. This risk is compounded when the person is overweight and a smoker. Also, non-steroidal anti-inflammatory medications, such as ibuprofen, and acetaminophen, may contribute to elevated blood pressure in susceptible women. However, acetominophen does not increase blood pressure in men.

African American women are more likely to have high blood pressure, especially earlier in life. The reason for this difference is not known.

Unfortunately, hypertension does not have a cure at this time, but it can be treated and brought under control by medication and lifestyle modifications. Aerobic conditioning can cause a significant improvement in blood pressure. Some studies have shown that up to 30% of those with mild hypertension who become physically conditioned can give up medications. For those who are overweight, as little as a ten pound weight loss can bring mild elevations of blood pressure into normal range.

In the past, the treatment of hypertension was not as aggressive and the recommendation was to slowly decrease the blood pressure. The latest recommendation for treatment of hypertension is to start early and to bring down the blood pressure to the normal acceptable range as fast as possible. There are times that blood pressure may be resistant to treatment, and further work-up may be needed at a hypertension specialty clinic.

Have your blood pressure checked by your physician and keep a log of the results.

High Blood Cholesterol (Hyperlipidemia/ Dyslipidemia)

> **Fast Fact**
> Half of all heart attacks occur in people with normal cholesterol levels.

High cholesterol is the second most common risk factor for heart disease. Again, as women get older, the risk of developing hyperlipidemia increases. Before menopause, women are usually protected by high levels of C-HDL (good cholesterol). Endogenous estrogen in the female body increases the level of this protective particle until menopause.

Cholesterol can be affected by genetics and diet. Since the hereditary factor cannot be altered yet, lifestyle modification including diet and exercise, and at times medication, are the ways to treat and effectively control high cholesterol.

Elevated total cholesterol, low density lipoprotein-C (bad cholesterol) and triglycerides, and low high density lipoprotein-C (good cholesterol) are known risk factors for coronary artery disease in women. In the past, the emphasis was on the ratios of the bad to good cholesterol. Nowadays, we know that the absolute numbers are more important and it is imperative for both women and men to know their numbers. A lipid panel is done to measure your total cholesterol, the good and the bad cholesterol, and triglycerides.

Triglycerides respond to reduction in overall calorie intake, weight loss and decrease in intake of sweets and alcohol. Fish oil and niacin are very effective treatments for high triglycerides. Patients with diabetes usually have a harder time managing this number.

Unfortunately, many of the clinical studies addressing cholesterol treatments have included an under-representation of women. More clinical trials are needed to address the effect of lipid lowering therapy on primary prevention of high cholesterol in women. Primary prevention means that the drug is used to prevent coronary artery events including heart attacks and death.

Cholesterol lowering can be achieved with either drugs or diet. At this time, most of the available information on the outcomes is based on the class of medications called statins. Few studies have looked at the effects of dietary and non-statin interventions on clinical outcomes.

What are the guidelines for acceptable cholesterol levels?

The American Heart Association
1. Total cholesterol

Total cholesterol should be less than 200 mg/dl. Some women attribute their high cholesterol level to their high C-HDL (good cholesterol) level. However, regardless of high C-HDL levels, the accepted absolute total cholesterol number remains at 200 mg/dl. If C-HDL is subtracted from the total cholesterol level, the value that is obtained is called the non-HDL level and it should be less than 130 mg/dl.

2. LDL cholesterol (the "bad cholesterol")

The level for the bad cholesterol has gone down over the years and a level of less than 130 mg/dl is considered good. The optimal level is less than 100 mg/dl which is enforced for patients with known heart disease or diabetics. However, new studies have pushed the low number even lower. For now, the patients with very high risks and known heart disease will benefit from an LDL level of less than 70 mg/dl.

3. HDL cholesterol (the "good cholesterol")

The good cholesterol should be over 50 mg/dl in women. Levels of HDL-C above 60 mg/dl are considered heart protective.

4. Triglycerides

The acceptable level for triglycerides is <150 mg/dl. Higher levels have been shown to increase the risk for heart disease in women.

Alternative guidelines based on EBCT coronary calcium scores

The Orange County Heart Institute has been working with EBCT heart scan technology for many years. We have found this to be a very reasonable, and indeed more scientific approach to cholesterol management. EBCT heart scans for coronary calcium (think of coronary calcium as the same thing as plaque or hardening of the arteries) have been shown to be a very effective tool to determine who should have their cholesterol treated. The coronary calcium reflects the effects of all your risk factors on your arteries and thus tells you the amount of atherosclerosis that you have in your coronary arteries. Based on the quantity of calcium, we also determine how vigorously to lower the cholesterol. (EBCT heart scans are discussed in more detail in Chapter 1.)

Smoking

There is no such thing as social smoking. If you smoke, you are increasing your risk for an array of diseases. Nothing good comes out of smoking, except shorter life filled with heart disease, lung disease and cancer. Women who smoke do not have the same protection from their female hormones as their non-smoking counterparts.

One in five women smokes and on average will die about fourteen and half years earlier than female nonsmokers. The risk of cigarette smoking is shown to be equivalent to the risk associated with weighing about 92 pounds more than your non-smoking counterpart. The risk for heart disease increases two to four times when one smokes. Smoking is the third most common risk factor for heart disease and the number one cause of premature death in this country.

However, the good news is you can decrease your risks and live a healthier life by quitting today. After one year of being cigarette-free, your excess risk of heart disease is reduced by about half. The risk continues to decrease over the next 10 to 15 years such that after 15 years, your risk is similar to a non-smoker.

Unfortunately, statistics show that more female teenagers, especially white females in high school, are smoking, despite the overall drop in smoking since 1965.

Smoking affects heart disease by causing fatty buildups in the heart and other arteries in the body, hence, increasing the risk of stroke as well. Smoking can increase blood pressure, decrease the good cholesterol (HDL), and decrease exercise tolerance. Therefore, not only can smoking directly increase the risk of heart disease, but can dramatically magnify the deleterious effects of other risk factors. As with hypertension, combined use of birth control pills and smoking places women at a higher risk for heart disease.

Cigar and pipe smoking is shown to increase the risk for heart disease, but not as much as cigarette smoking. This has been attributed to the possibility of inhaling less with cigars and pipes, but more studies need to be done.

Women and men who are exposed to secondhand smoke have a higher risk of developing heart disease as well. About 35,000 people a year die from heart disease due to second-hand smoke, also known as environmental tobacco smoke.

Diabetes

A fasting blood sugar level over 126 mg/dl is considered to define diabetes, a very serious disease which slowly debilitates many organs in the body. In the past, women were thought to be at higher risk for heart disease than men when they had diabetes, but some studies have refuted that claim. We do know that diabetic women or men are at higher risk for having heart disease even when their blood sugar is under control. A woman with diabetes is twice as likely to have a major cardiac event than one without diabetes. Those with diabetes also tend to have more "silent" heart attacks. Somehow, diabetes affects the nerve sensation from the heart which makes symptoms an even less reliable indicator of disease. For this reason, diabetic patients need careful, lifelong screening to detect heart disease.

Obesity

Obesity is an epidemic in this country and an emerging and serious problem in children as well. It is one of the major risk factors for heart disease and is closely related to diabetes and physical inactivity. Obesity increases the strain on the heart and increases the risk by influencing other risk factors. With our fast food diet and sedentary lifestyle, we are placing ourselves at a very high risk for developing a condition that can be prevented. Body Mass Index (BMI) is one way of knowing whether one is overweight or obese and it can be roughly calculated at home: weight in pounds times 705, divided by height in inches, divided by height in inches.

If the BMI is less than 25, then it is within the acceptable range, if it's over 30, then you are obese, and in between is considered overweight. You also do not want to have a very low number (lower than 18.5) which places you into the underweight category.

It is also important to know your waist circumference since a waist measurement of over 35 inches places a woman at higher risk for heart disease. Studies have shown that fat in the abdominal area is more predictive of having heart disease later in life. Therefore, fat around the stomach is worse that fat around the hips, so it's better to look like a pear than an apple. Even losing as little as 10 to 12 pounds can decrease one's risk for developing heart disease.

You may have heard about metabolic syndrome which means

having a combination of some the above risk factors. A woman with metabolic syndrome is at high risk for having heart disease in her life. A patient has metabolic syndrome if she has three or more of the following risks:

- waist circumference more than 35 inches
- triglycerides more than 150 mg/dl
- HDL less than 50 mg/dl
- blood pressure more than 130/85 mm Hg
- fasting glucose level more than 110 mg/dl

Physical Inactivity

As people age, they are less likely to be physically active. Exercising reduces the risk for diabetes, obesity, high blood pressure and high cholesterol. However, about 39% of adults in this country do not exercise. Studies show that physical inactivity can increase the risk of heart disease as much 50%. It is important to know that any type of physical activity is encouraged and can be beneficial.

The American Heart Association recommends a moderate-intensity activity at least 30 minutes on most, and preferably, all days of the week.

Is stress a risk factor?

We know that there is a relationship between stress and cardiovascular diseases, however, we do not yet know if stress is an independent risk factor. Women under stress are more likely to smoke and overeat. We do know that smoking is a risk factor, and overeating can contribute to high blood pressure, high cholesterol, obesity and diabetes, all known risk factors for heart disease. Everyone has some level of stress. What we do want people to do is to find out how to best manage everyday stress and seek help when necessary to avoid the harmful consequences of stress.

A recent study demonstrated that men who were stressed by a controlling wife tended to have more hardening of the coronary arteries, whereas women who felt hostility from their spouses tended to have more hardening of the arteries. A controlling husband seemed not to adversely affect the women's hearts (at least in this study). Recent studies also show that chronic job stress contributes to elevation of the LDL (bad) cholesterol and contributes to the development of the metabolic syndrome.

Emerging Risk Factors
1. *Lp (a)*
2. *Homocysteine*
3. *C-reactive protein (CRP)*
4. *Low subtype HDL2b*
5. *Small- size LDL cholesterol particle*
6. *Bacterial infections*

The above risk factors have been under study over the past decade. They can be identified with an Advanced Lipid Panel your physician may order. Recent studies are postulating the need to examine more novel risk factors for women. Not all patients need to have an advanced cholesterol panel, but there are times that a patient may not respond to regular cholesterol therapy, or they may have borderline cholesterol levels with strong family history, or they are at a particularly high risk for heart disease. In those instances, a more detailed lipid panel may help the physician to better tailor patients' treatments. The Advanced Lipid Panel becomes especially useful when a patient develops significant coronary disease at a younger than expected age. This may be seen when a person gets an EBCT heart scan to look for coronary calcium (plaque). If the patient has an unusually high level of coronary calcium, it is imperative to search for all possible corrective causes and risk factors. These patients often have one of the above mentioned risk factors, and once identified, proper medical treatment can be instituted.

1. Lp(a)—Lipoprotein – (a)
The level of this small protein is determined by our genetic make-up. Two recent studies in women confirm that an Lp(a) level of more than 30, doubles the risk of heart attack and stroke.

If the level of Lp(a) is more than 65, then the risk is 67% higher. Lp(a) is thought to contribute to inflammation and clot formation in the arteries. It attaches to the bad cholesterol (LDL) and increases the risk for plaque formation in the artery walls. It does not change with diet since genetics has a role in its level. In general, niacin in high doses (more than 1000 mg per day) is the most effective treatment.

2. Homocysteine

There is still a controversy about whether high levels of homocysteine need aggressive treatment. However, for high risks patients the trend is to treat them if their homocysteine level is increased. Homocysteine level goes up when there is a lack of certain vitamins or enzymes responsible for metabolism of amino acids. Amino acids are building blocks for protein. In general, vitamin B_6, vitamin B_{12} and folic acid are the most effective treatment.

3. CRP (C-Reactive Protein)

Inflammation plays a role in the hardening of arteries. When inflammation is present and at a high level, some proteins are formed in the blood as an indication of the inflammatory process. CRP is one of them. This marker becomes useful in patients who are at high risk for heart disease and the physician is not convinced that the current treatment is optimal. Also, when the cholesterol levels are not very elevated, CRP can guide the physician in deciding whether to treat the patient with diet or medication. In this case, a borderline elevated cholesterol and a high CRP level might warrant treatment of the cholesterol. The statin class of cholesterol medications and aspirin are the most effective treatment for arterial inflammation which causes the CRP to increase. It is important to know that different inflammations in the body, such as arthritis, can also increase the level of CRP, so the cardiologist will look at the range the CRP falls into in order to correlate it to heart disease rather than to other entities.

4. Low Subtype HDL2b

In recent years, it has been shown that the good cholesterol (HDL-C) can be broken down into smaller units. Not all of these sub-units are the protective ones, as some studies show. HDL-C plays a very important role in protecting women from heart disease and heart attacks. It is usually higher in women than men because of the effect of the endogenous estrogen. We do know that HDL has the job of cleaning the walls of the arteries by removing cholesterol plaques. Of the different sub-units of HDL, only the HDL2b is the true cleaning sub-unit. It can be measured when an advanced lipid panel is ordered. Advanced lipid panels may be done in patients with other risk factors and especially in those with a strong family history. If it is found that a low HDL2b is the cause of the atherosclerosis, niacin is the most effective treatment.

5. Small Size LDL Cholesterol

Not only is the level of LDL-C (bad cholesterol) important as a risk factor, but also the **size** of the molecule. LDL-C is responsible for forming plaque buildup in the walls of the arteries. It is one of the strongest risk factors for heart disease. Therefore, high risk patients may need a more thorough look at their cholesterol levels to assess the size of their LDL-C. The smaller molecule size of LDL increases the risk of plaque buildup. The statin class of cholesterol medications are very effective in lowering the total LDL cholesterol, but do not change the LDL size. Niacin is the most effective medication to change small and dense LDL to larger and less dangerous LDL particles.

6. Bacterial Infections: Do they cause or affect heart disease?

The most studied bacteria found in the plaques of some patients with heart disease are *Chlamydia pneumonia*. This bacteria can cause pneumonia and bronchitis. No studies have shown a cause and effect between coronary artery disease and bacterial infection. Furthermore, antibiotic treatments for Chlamydia (short term or long term) have not prevented further heart attacks in patients with heart disease or previous heart attacks. There are no recommendations for treating this bacteria at this time.

Remember, keep a copy of your lipid panel for reference.

3

Chest Pain and Heart Attacks

Chest pain is the most misused word in cardiology. Chest pain is a very convenient word to use, but most discomfort that may be heart related is almost never described as "pain" by the patient. Even when a patient is having a heart attack, they will rarely describe the sensation as a pain, it is often described as a discomfort or ache. The medical term for a heart related attack is *angina pectoris* or just *angina*.

Angina is a specific term that refers to any discomfort that is due to a narrowed coronary artery that is restricting blood flow to the heart muscle. The chest discomfort of angina is usually described as a pressure sensation, or squeezing, or ache, tightness, burning, or a dull discomfort. To cause this discomfort, your coronary artery has to have a narrowing of at least 60 % to 70 % before there is a restriction of blood flow to the heart. The medical term for the state that exists when there is a decrease in blood flow to the heart, it is called *ischemia*. However, the symptom is called angina.

Angina in women may have different characteristics than in men. Often in women, instead of a chest discomfort, there is exertional fatigue, unusual breathlessness, indigestion (especially with exertion), jaw ache, unusual sweating with activity and pain in the shoulders. All these symptoms can be early warning signs for women of inadequate blood flow to their heart. Of course, the classic symptoms of chest pressure, ache or squeezing sensation in the mid chest or left side, which may radiate to the left, right or both arms, can certainly be an indication of a heart problem, as it often is in men. However, the most characteristic quality is that the symptom comes on with some type of exertion, like walking, stair climbing, doing laundry, or lifting, and then the sensation resolves slowly when the activity stops.

How can I tell the discomfort is not my heart?

If the chest pain is very sharp, very brief for no more than a few seconds at a time, or if it gets worse or better by pushing on the area of the chest, shoulders or upper arms, or turning, or moving the arm or chest area, or deep breathing, then it is unlikely the pain is from the heart. The pain is most likely from the chest wall, muscle or ribs. Even so, try to remember what it felt like, where it was located at the time, and the duration of the pain or discomfort.

Does it radiate to another body part? What will trigger the pain? What will relieve the pain? Are other symptoms associated with the pain such as shortness of breath, sweating (diaphoresis), nausea, lightheadedness? The ability to describe the discomfort to your doctor will determine what type of testing will be done.

What tests are needed to determine if the discomfort is angina?

Diagnostic tests for chest pain include a simple treadmill test, a stress echocardiogram, or a nuclear stress test, EBCT scans or noninvasive CT angiograms. More advanced evaluations would include a cardiac catheterization and coronary angiogram. These tests are described in detail in Chapter 1. Remember that a doctor needs to evaluate any chest pain of new onset.

What is the difference between an episode of angina and a heart attack?

Angina is an early warning sign of a heart attack. Angina is discomfort from the heart due to temporary decrease in blood flow to the heart. However, the decrease in blood flow is of short duration (usually less than 15 minutes), and therefore, there is *no damage to the heart*. If any of the angina symptoms lasts more than 15 minutes you may be having a heart attack! The difference between angina and a heart attack is that with angina the blood flow is not enough to meet the needs of the heart so discomfort occurs, but the duration is short and there is no heart damage. A heart attack means there is complete obstruction of blood flow to the heart and heart muscle damage is occurring. If the pattern of angina changes, for instance, the discomfort lasts longer, is more intense, is occurring with less and less exertion, or occurs at rest, this means that the narrowed artery is becoming rapidly more constricted and a heart attack is imminent.

A heart attack saga

The middle-aged business executive described her heart attack as if she had been punched in both shoulders. Another woman was a 40-year-old teacher who had no chest or shoulder pain at all. She described her heart attack symptoms as more of an ache in her upper back, along with indigestion-like symptoms in lower chest area. Then there was the case of a women who felt no ache or pain, just an uncomfortable feeling in the pit of the stomach. Three different presenting symptoms, yet all three were diagnosed with heart attacks.

The less dramatic symptoms that women often experience during a heart attack along with the common perception that heart disease is a man's disease, often leads to a delay in treatment when women are seen in a an emergency room. The delay in treatment, especially for women under 50, though it true for older women as well, explains in part the reason for a higher mortality rates for women with heart attacks. Most women simply don't have the severe crushing chest pain that is so characteristic of men. In addition, frequently even when women develop the male-typical symptoms, they have a tendency to deny those symptoms as heart related and ignore timely treatment.

Early Warning Signs

In a recent study of 515 women who suffered heart attacks, 95% of them reported that they had unusual, new or different symptoms for a month or so prior to their heart attacks.

Major symptoms reported prior to the heart attack
Seventy - unusual fatigue
Forty-eight - sleep disturbance
Forty-two - shortness of breath
Thirty-nine - indigestion
Thirty-five - anxiety

Major acute symptoms during the heart attack
Fifty-eight - shortness of breath
Fifty-five - weakness
Forty-three - unusual fatigue
Forty-two - cold sweat
Thirty-nine - dizziness

What to do if you think it is a heart attack

If any of the suggested above symptoms lasts more than 15 minutes, especially if accompanied with profuse sweating, weakness, shortness of breath and nausea–you could very likely be having a heart attack. Get immediate medical attention. Remember indigestion type symptoms can often be actually heart related. If belching relieves the symptoms only slightly, don't be fooled. It could still be heart related.

Should these symptoms strike, take an adult aspirin immediately and call 911 or less desirably have someone drive you to the nearest emergency room. Don't drive yourself; you are putting yourself and others at risk.

What to expect on arrival at the emergency room

State clearly and very directly that you think you are having symptoms of a heart attack. Demand to be seen immediately by a nurse or physician. Don't be put off. It is your body and you have every right to expect the best diagnosis available. Don't minimize your symptoms to the health care provider. This could delay your treatment and medical evaluation.

Expect to have an ECG within 5 to 10 minutes upon arrival. Demand it! Although the ECG can be normal in 50% of the people having a heart attack evaluation, the ECG is a crucial first diagnostic test. If your ECG is abnormal, it will accelerate the diagnosis and often guide the treatment course. There is a certain characteristic change on the ECG, called the *ST segment,* which is examined for certain abnormalities. If the ST segment is elevated, this signifies a total occlusion or blockage of the artery. When this occurs, the usual treatment is the administration of clot-busting drugs, blood thinners or perhaps an emergency coronary angiogram and angioplasty. The emergency room physician and cardiologist will make these decisions for you.

Fast Fact
Do not minimize your symptoms when you arrive in the emergency room. State that you think you may be having a heart attack. Request an ECG and to be seen immediately by a nurse or doctor.

State of the art treatment for a heart attack with ST segment elevation on a standard 12 lead ECG:

Perform emergency coronary angiography and implant an intra-coronary stent in the blocked artery. This should usually be done with in 90 minutes upon arriving in the emergency room. This requires of course, that the hospital you go to has the appropriate catheterization lab and cardiologists available. This also requires that you have no contraindications to the procedure. Only trained cardiologists can make this decision for you,

Blood tests are drawn soon after arrival, usually within 15 minutes on arrival. These blood tests measure cardiac *enzymes.* Cardiac enzymes are chemicals that are released into the blood stream from the heart muscle if it is damaged by a heart attack. Often cardiac enzymes are not released into the bloodstream for 2 to 3 hours after the start of a heart attack; therefore, subsequent cardiac enzymes are measured 4 to 6 hours later.

You will be given a chewable aspirin. The aspirin interrupts the blood platelets that are forming the clotting process in the coronary artery. Additional treatment consists of oxygen administered through nasal prongs, and if chest discomfort is still present, a nitroglycerin tablet or spray under the tongue to dilate the narrowed coronary artery to improve blood flow. Morphine is the routinely given intravenously if the chest discomfort persists despite the use of nitroglycerin.

When is a heart attack a heart attack?

Our understanding of the process of coronary insufficiency or ischemia (the process of decreased blood flow through the coronary arteries) has become more detailed and refined in the past several years. In a sense, not all heart attacks are the same. We now offer treatment that is now more precisely tailored to the underlying process that is occurring at the actual plaque. When angina symptoms quickly change in character, that is, the symptoms are much more intense, or prolonged or at rest, this is referred to as *unstable angina* or *acute coronary syndrome (ACS)*. The process at the plaque in the coronary artery that is causing the decrease in blood flow is referred to as the plaque becoming "unstable." By tailoring the treatment, the outcome and survival benefits are much improved. Still, it requires timely and immediate treatment.

When blood flow is reduced to the heart muscle by intermittent and recurring closure and opening of the coronary artery, the symptoms of angina become more prolonged, more intense and often will occur at rest. This is referred to as unstable angina and is a precursor to a full-blown heart attack. The ECG often shows minor T segment depression rather than the classical ST elevation as seen in the ECG of the classical full-blown heart attack. The significance of this is that the plaque that is narrowing and restricting the blood flow is now being plugged with platelet filled clots (so called "white clots"), these are best treated with drugs that inhibit platelets from sticking together in a cluster, forming a clot.

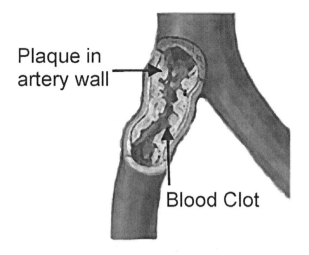

Plaque in artery wall

Blood Clot

They call these platelet inhibiting drugs, 2B, 3A inhibitors, some of the commonly used ones are *Integrellin* or *Aggrestat.* The cardiologist makes this determination whether to give these platelet inhibitors versus the clot-busting drugs called thrombolytics traditionally given for the full-blown heart attack. The cardiologist would also determine if and when a coronary angiogram should be done.

The "classical" heart attack *(myocardial infarction)* is the sudden closure of a coronary artery with cessation of arterial blood flow to a portion of the heart muscle. Acute heart attack strikes when a pre-existing buildup of lipids (fat) or plaque, is squeezed into a coronary artery and ruptures. The rupture of this fat-laden plaque stimulates platelets within the blood and causes them to clump and form a clot (thrombus). If the clot does not completely block (occlude) the vessel, then the patient in most cases experiences a pattern of severe, unstable, recurrent chest pain called unstable angina (acute coronary syndrome).

Should the clot completely occlude the vessel, without backup, which is collateral flow from other coronary arteries, you'll likely experiences severe chest pain that fails to ease with oxygen, rest, or nitroglycerin. Should the clot fail to dissolve and blood flow is not reestablished, permanent injury or heart muscle damage occurs.

When this happens, prolonged severe pain or pressure occurs, often with sweating, nausea and breathlessness. However, with about thirty percent or more cases, mostly women, the heart attack is silent or not even recognized by the patient. If it does cause discomfort, it may be soreness, a shortness of breath, or a feeling of indigestion. These silent heart attacks tend to be smaller in size and less severe.. They more often occur in those with diabetics, obesity, hypertension or smokers. We are not certain why diabetics are less likely to feel the pain of a heart attack; it is probably due to the neuropathy (chronic nerve damage) that often occurs due to diabetes. For women as well as men, acute myocardial infarction (acute MI) causes the death of the myocardium (heart muscle) following a coronary artery closure.

So, when is a heart attack a heart attack? Whenever there is heart muscle damage, there is a heart attack. Due to the ever more sensitive tests to detect even the smallest heart muscle damage, our definition of a heart attack is changing. The classical so called full blown heart attack with "ST segment elevation" can be quickly treated with an intra-coronary stent and result in almost undetectable damage to the heart, as little as seen in those with the unstable angina pattern. Even with the unstable angina pattern of symptoms, though not thought of as a classical heart attack, there probably is microscopic amounts of heart muscle damage. So depending on how long the blood flow is diminished, regardless of the underlying process, there can be small, medium and large heart attacks. The long term outcome from a heart attack depends on how much muscle is damaged. Quick recognition of symptoms and prompt treatment is essential to saving your life.

Plaque rupture and thrombus formation

It is not certain of the exact factors that come into play and cause a pre-existing coronary plaque to rupture and stimulate clot formation. There is growing evidence that inflammation of the lining of the artery leads to plaque rupture. What causes the inflammation is unclear. Certain irritants like smoking, high levels of blood fatty acids and possible infections are all implicated. Statin type cholesterol medications are given in patients with heart attacks or angina, or anyone with known coronary artery disease, because statins *stabilize* the plaque and reduce inflammation of the lining of the coronary lining even before they have any effect on cholesterol lowering. For whatever the reason, some plaques appear unstable are prone to rupture. This may happen as the fat content swells in the plaque and the thin fibrous cap that covers the plaque develops a tear. At that moment, there is a release of fatty material onto the surface of the plaque, into the opening of the artery. This material stimulates the cascade of clot formation. Blood platelets clump together, and then larger clots (thrombus) form.

If properly diagnosed, when a clot forms, drugs can be given that can dissolv the clot. TPA (*tissue plasminogen activator*), TNK, and streptokinase are the most commonly prescribed drugs to dissolve coronary thrombosis. These are only effective in re-storing blood flow in about 60 to 80 percent of the time. In addition, these drugs carry about a 1 in 1,000 risk of causing an intracerebral hemorrhage (bleeding in the brain). Even though the rare risk of intracerebral bleeding may occur, doctors feel that TPA is worth prescribing because it dissolves the coronary arterial clot, reducing the risk of extensive heart damage and possibly death.

The greatest opportunity of success comes with administration of thrombolytic drugs within two hours of the onset of chest pain or presumed thrombotic closure of the vessel. Fortunately, if these medications are given early on, there is an excellent chance of full recovery of the heart muscle. If the clot is dissolved within 2 to 6 hours, then partial recovery of the heart muscle occurs, yet often there will remain some persistent heart muscle weakness of varying degree. After 6 hours without restoring blood flow, it is doubtful that the heart muscle will recover. However, reperfusion (reestablishing blood flow) can help prevent enlargement of the heart and the development of severe muscle damage which can lead to congestive heart failure. Time is heart muscle. The sooner you recognize that your symptoms may be heart related, the sooner you get effective treatment in the emergency room, the less likely you will have significant heart damage.

The trend presently is to intervene with emergency angiography and opening the artery with coronary angioplasty and insertion of an intra-coronary stent. The decision to administer clot busting medications and or performing emergency coronary stenting is often a complex decision made by an experienced interventional cardiologist.

The underlying cause of heart attacks

Coronary artery disease (CAD) is the underlying problem that leads to a heart attack (MI). CAD is the process where plaques (or lesions) develop within the coronary arterial wall. These plaques are composed of fats, fiber, and calcium that cause thickening of the arterial wall and narrowing of the channel through which blood flows. They commonly call this "hardening of the arteries" (or atherosclerosis).

Though CAD may start in young people, it is more likely manifests itself in older patients. The age at which hardening of the arteries first occurs is dependent on the amount of "risk factors" a person has.

Can a heart attack occur if the arteries are normal?

There are rare occasions when a heart attack can occur when the coronary arteries are free of plaque. The most notable cause is severe spasm of the coronary artery in response to some severe stress, for instance, after an argument or form taking a strong stimulant like cocaine. The artery temporarily squeezes down and reduces blood flow long enough to cause heart muscle damage, then the artery eventually relaxes and resumes its normal caliber. These patients respond to medications that relax the artery, like calcium channel blocker class of drugs, plus aspirin as well cholesterol medicines and fish oil which help reduce inflammation in the lining of the artery.

Another scenario of a heart attack in a patient with normal coronary arteries occurs when a clot lodges in the artery. Usually there is some underlying clotting disorder or exposure to some environmental factor that promotes clotting, like tobacco or stimulants like cocaine. Aspirin, Plavix and sometimes warfarin (coumadin) are needed to prevent future heart attacks in these particular cases.

A case of stress and the heart:

J.V. was a healthy 42-year-old female with no risk factors other than a mild elevation of her cholesterol. She was not on any medications. Shortly after a very intense argument with a neighbor, she had a severe tightness and pressure across her entire chest radiating somewhat into her back. The discomfort persisted as a severe ache for less than half an hour. Thereafter, a low-grade chest ache remained.

Almost 24 hours later, the low grade discomfort persisted and she was seen in our office. A stress echocardiogram was attempted but the chest discomfort increased in less than a minute. The echocardiogram showed a discrete segment of the anterior wall and the inferior wall of the left ventricle (the main pumping chamber of the heart) were not contracting normally. There was evidence of damage to the heart muscle. She was brought emergently to the hospital. An invasive coronary angiogram confirmed what was seen on the echocardiogram. The front and bottom of the hear walls were not contracting normally. There had been a small heart attack. Interestingly, the coronary arteries were perfectly normal. No evidence of a clot, no ongoing spasm or tear in the arteries. She did not require a stent or PTCA. Cardiac enzymes confirmed the fact hat she did have a heart attack (heart damage). The assumption was that the adrenaline surge during the argument produced severe spasm of at least two of the three coronary arteries since the heart muscle function and damage occurred in two different artery distributions. She was placed on a calcium channel blocker to prevent spasm, aspirin to prevent any potential clotting and a statin to lower her cholesterol and for its anti-inflammatory properties. She was also placed on fish oil for its anti-clotting, anti-inflammatory properties and its potential to make the artery walls more flexible. L-arginine was also added for its potential to from nitric oxide in the artery wall and relax the artery wall. Three weeks later, a stress echocardiogram was entirely normal. No evidence whatsoever of any heart muscle damage! She has now returned to a normal active lifestyle. What was unique about this particular situation was that her spasm was severe enough to affect at least two arteries of the heart, since the front and bottom (inferior wall) of the heart were both damaged, and each wall is supplied by a different artery. She has had a full recovery and we expect a very low probability of future occurrences.

Risk factors for coronary artery disease include:

- Cigarette smoking
- High blood pressure
- Family history / genetics
- Diabetes
- High LDL ("bad" cholesterol)
- Low HDL ("good" cholesterol)
- Age
- Male sex

These risk factors were discussed in more detail in chapter 2.

In summary

As the plaques first arise in the coronary arterial wall, there are no symptoms. If the plaque ruptures, then a heart attack strikes with closure of the artery by a blood clot.

It is vital that younger women realize that they are as much at risk for a heart attack as men. This is a difficult medical problem for women in our culture. Educating women about heart disease is the most potent weapon in reducing death from heart attacks. Early detection of heart disease saves lives. Recognizing the symptoms of heart disease is the crucial first step in seeking rapid and effective treatment that may save *your* life.

4

Treating Chest Pain
Without Surgery

Nancy felt an uncomfortable pressure in her left shoulder for about two weeks. It seemed to occur only during her lunch break when she went for her usual 20 minute walk. She started her walking program after vowing to lose the 30 pounds she gained earlier in the year. Her weekends were free of discomfort even though she continued her walk, albeit in the mornings before breakfast. The third weekend, out of routine, she had breakfast, then went for her walk. It was the coolest morning of the new fall season. She felt the same disconcerting shoulder ache that she had noticed while walking at work. This time however, she felt slightly short of breath. She cut her walk short.

The following week, she saw her physician who ordered a stress echocardiogram. It was abnormal. We recommended an invasive coronary angiogram which showed a 60% narrowing in the coronary artery in the back of the heart. We felt that she could be managed medically. She was started on 81 mg. of aspirin, a statin type of cholesterol lowering drug and a weight loss program. After she adjusted to her medications, she entered a supervised exercise program. Over the subsequent six months she lost 20 pounds, was free of chest pain and was back to her lunchtime walks, this time before eating. A repeat stress echocardiogram was significantly improved and she continued with weight loss, exercise and medications.

Angina

As mentioned in the previous chapters, angina is a specific term that refers to chest discomfort. It isn't a disease, but rather a symptom of decreased blood flow to the heart; a heart attack means that you have actually sustained damage to the heart muscle.

For heart muscle damage to occur, the heart muscle needs to be deprived of adequate blood for about 15 minutes or more. You are not having "mini heart attacks" with each brief angina episode. It should also be remembered that some patients have heart attacks but no recognizable symptoms. These so called *silent heart attacks* occur more frequently in patients with hypertension or diabetes. It's not clear why those with hypertension may experience silent heart attacks, but it is thought that nerve damage diabetes causes might make diabetics less likely to experience angina.

Fast Fact
Women tend to have angina more often at rest or due to stress than men. Men seem to have more angina with exertion.

A patient with chronic angina is more likely to have a heart attack than a person who has no known heart disease and does not have angina. However, we can greatly reduce or totally eliminate the episodes of angina, and significantly reduce the risk of a heart attack. Many patients with chronic angina can live fairly normal lives and fairly normal life spans when carefully monitored by their physicians.

Chronic angina is typical angina that has been occurring for months or years. It is considered *stable angina* when it occurs in a predictable manner; for instance, if the discomfort occurs with relatively the same amount of exertion, or if the angina is always felt as a chest tightness that radiates to the left arm. If the intensity is about the same with each episode, the duration is the same after stopping activity, and the same quantity of nitroglycerin relieves the angina, these are all characteristics of *stable angina.*

Unstable angina is any change in *intensity, duration, quality or the need for nitroglycerine.* If the character of the angina changes, that is, if it now radiates to both arms and to the jaw, then the angina is actually worsening because the artery is becoming more constricted. The angina is no longer *stable.* This change in pattern needs to be reported to the physician immediately because it usually means that the plaque in the artery responsible for the angina in the first place, is now progressing rapidly and becoming unstable. A narrowed section of the artery which was, say, a stable 80% narrowing, is now quickly narrowing and complete closure of the artery with a subsequent heart attack is imminent. (See Chapter 2 on acute coronary syndrome.)

There are a few conditions that can change the pattern of stable angina and not *necessarily mean that the plaque is changing:*

• After eating, angina may occur with less than the usual amount of exertion. For instance, if you can normally walk two miles before getting angina, however, after eating a meal the angina may occur within a mile of walking. The explanation is that the heart has to work harder to digest the food and meet the needs of the muscles during walking. Since the narrowed coronary artery can only supply a limited amount of blood to the heart muscle, angina will occur more readily.

• Exposure to extremes of cold or heat put increased demands on the heart to work harder. Angina then may occur more readily, or last longer, or be more intense.

• If your body is retaining excess fluid (as in mild congestive heart failure), you may get angina after lying supine in bed while asleep. The explanation is that the excess fluid during the daytime hours when you are sitting or standing, is pulled into the legs or abdominal cavity. While lying down, gravity is no longer keeping the fluid away from the heart. The excess fluid reenters the blood stream, travels back to the heart, overstretches it and increases its workload.

• Anemia or thyroid problems, both easily diagnosed with routine blood tests, can sometimes cause a significant increase in angina symptoms.

• Sometimes switching to a generic brand of medication may cause stable symptoms to become more severe.

Medical versus surgical treatment

The decision to treat a patient with medications instead of coronary bypass surgery or stents is complex. Some of the factors are directly related to the heart itself; others to conditions in the body that may make surgery riskier than medical treatment.

Conditions related to the heart that influence treatment include:

• The extent of the blockages in the coronary arteries as seen on a coronary angiogram. Are the blockages diffuse through out the artery, or discrete in one segment of the artery? Are blockages at the beginning of the arteries or at the end? Are they at a branch point where two arteries divide? How healthy is the heart function, i.e., is the heart pumping function (ejection fraction) normal or reduced?

• Exercise capacity on a treadmill stress test. When do symptoms develop during the exercise period and how abnormal does the EKG, echocardiogram or nuclear scan become during exercise?

• How often and severe are the angina symptoms during daily activities?

Non heart-related conditions the cardiologist considers include:

• Age of the patient. There are "old" 80-year-olds and "young" 80-year-olds. This "physiological age," believe it or not, is often very important in the outcome of surgeries, often more so than the chronological age.

• Patient's lifestyle, occupation and, of course, desire for surgery versus medications. For instance, a pilot may be more likely to retain her license if she had coronary bypass surgery.

• What is the condition of the other organs of the body? Is the lung function abnormal due to smoking or some other chronic lung condition? Is the kidney function normal or reduced? Is the liver functioning normally? Are there other conditions like ulcers in the stomach or duodenum which may lead to bleeding problems if surgery is performed?

• Does the patient have diabetes, high blood pressure, cancer, or blood problems that may lead to excess bleeding or clotting problems?

• Are there problems with other arteries or veins that will make surgery more difficult or less likely to have a successful outcome?

Medications for Stable Angina

Medications to prevent progression of plaque

Cholesterol lowering medications are essential for any person with angina, even if the cholesterol level is normal. Since angina is usually caused by plaque build up in the arteries, it is essential to undertake all measures to prevent plaque progression, not only in the coronary artery which may be the cause of the angina, but the other coronary arteries which are also susceptible to plaque formation.

• Aspirin is essential to prevent clot formation at the plaque which can lead to a heart attack. Doses range from 81 mgs to 325 mgs per day.

• (Note:) Exercise, weight loss, control of high blood pressure, control of diabetes and congestive heart failure are all essential to effectively treating chronic angina.

Medications to treat angina symptoms:

Four different classes of medications are available to treat angina.

1. Beta blockers
2. Nitroglycerin compounds
3. Calcium channel blockers
4. Ranexa

The physician will choose among these medications based on a number of factors. For instance, some of the medications have a side effect of slowing the heart rate (beta blockers, verapamil and diltiazem). If the patient has a slow heart rate to begin with, these medications may be used only at low doses or only if other medications are ineffective. Contrarily, these same medications may be a first line choice if the patient is also prone to certain type of abnormal rapid heart rhythms (atrial fibrillation or supraventricular tachycardias). Beta blockers and calcium channel blockers also treat high blood pressure as well as angina, so these medications might be a better first line choice than long acting nitroglycerin.

As you can see, the decision on which type of medications to use can be quite complex and will be decided only after your doctor has thoroughly reviewed your condition.

Fast Fact
Due to a natural tendency toward more leg swelling than men, women tend to tolerate beta-blockers or nitrates better than calcium channel blockers.

---

1. Beta Blocking Compounds

Beta blockers are a cornerstone in the treatment of angina, not only because they are very effective in preventing angina that occurs with exertion (the most common type of angina), but also because only beta blockers have been shown to decrease the chance of a second heart attack as well as prolong survival.

Beta blockers are so called because they inhibit or block the nerve receptors, called beta receptors, on the heart, blood vessels and other organs. These receptors are called *beta*$_1$ and *beta*$_2$ receptors and are found in different proportion in various organs. The various types of beta blockers inhibit these receptors in various proportions. The receptors are stimulated by adrenaline-like compounds, so beta blockers essentially blunt or block the effect of adrenaline on the various organs. The effect is slowing of the heart rate, decreasing the force of contraction of the heart, and lowering blood pressure. These actions reduce the work load on the heart, essentially allowing the heart to function with less oxygen being delivered to the contracting heart muscle. Therefore, even though the artery is narrowed, the needs of the heart are now matched to the oxygen available, so angina is less likely to occur.

Types of Beta Blockers

The different types of beta blockers have different potential to block the different beta receptors, and therefore have slightly different benefits and drawbacks. If both receptors are blocked equally, the drugs are called *non-selective beta blockers.* If they tend to block primarily the beta receptors in the heart (beta$_1$), they are called *selective beta blockers*. Most can be taken once or twice per day. Some come in delayed release formulations for patients who have angina on awakening in the morning. You take these medications at bedtime and they are fully effective by the time you awake in the morning.

• Selective beta blockers primarily affect the heart and are therefore referred to as cardioselective. They tend to have fewer side effects because they have less effect on the beta$_2$ receptors that influence lung function, diabetes, peripheral blood flow in the legs and arms, and receptors in the brain that control mood. Metoprolol and atenolol are the two most common.

• Nonselective beta blockers have a potentially higher side effect profile because they affect all beta receptors; therefore, they are more likely to make asthma worse or affect diabetes control. Propranolol is the oldest and most commonly used drug in this class.

• Stimulating beta blockers tend to cause less slowing of the resting heart rate, but otherwise function as other beta blockers during exercise or stress by blunting the heart rate response and the contractile force of the heart. Pindolol and acebutolol are the two most common drugs in this category.

• Alpha receptor/beta blockers have the additional benefit of dilating blood vessels by inhibiting alpha receptors. This may be additionally helpful in patients with congestive heart failure. Carvedilol and labetolol are the two most common alpha receptor/beta blockers.

Side Effects
• Nervous system: depression, fatigue, nightmares, difficulty thinking.
   • Lungs: worsening of asthma, bronchial constriction.
   • Extremities: cold extremities, pain in the legs with walking in patients with poor circulation.

2. Nitroglycerin Compounds (Nitrates)

Nitroglycerin (NTG) compounds all have the common action of dilating arteries, predominantly the coronary arteries. They therefore relieve angina by increasing blood flow to the heart muscle. Their side effects are mainly related to the same action. By dilating blood vessels in the head they can cause headaches, dizziness and flushing sensations. The main difference between the various nitrate drugs is related to the onset and duration of action.

• Nitroglycerin sublingual. The sublingual form is commonly a tablet, but a spray is also available. Both have onset of action in one to five minutes and last about 15 minutes to one-half hour. They are used mainly to stop an attack of angina if the discomfort does not resolve on its own in four to five minutes. You may also take the tablet if a particular active routine causes angina. For instance, if walking to the car routinely causes angina, you can prevent it by taking NTG sublingually five to ten minutes before. The tablets deteriorate in six months and are best stored sealed in a bottle away from moisture and light. The spray form is stable for about two years.
• Long acting nitroglycerin: isosorbide dinitrate (ISDN) and isosorbide mononitrate (ISMN). Both have onset in about 15 to 30 minutes. The ISDN lasts three to six hours and is taken twice

per day. The ISMN lasts about six to eight hours and is taken once per day.

• Transdermal nitroglycerin. The patch acts in about 30 minutes and lasts about 14 to 15 hours. The nitroglycerin seeps through a membrane in the patch into the skin, then into the blood stream. You can place the patch anywhere on the upper body, not necessarily over the heart. Usually it is applied in the morning and removed at bedtime to prevent a tolerance build up to the nitroglycerin. However, some patients develop angina when the patch is removed, and in such cases, the patch is left on 24 hours before changing.

Side Effects

Headache, flushing, palpitations and dizziness are the most common side effects. Fainting can occur due to lowering of the blood pressure, especially if you are slightly dehydrated, if the weather is hot or if alcohol has been ingested. As a rule of thumb, it is better to sit down while taking the NTG sublingually. Then when it is time to stand, do so slowly. If lightheadedness does occur, sit or lie down immediately and the symptoms usually pass in five to ten minutes.

3. Calcium Channel Blockers

Calcium channel blockers are a versatile class of drugs used to treat high blood pressure, certain types of abnormal heart rhythms and angina. They are effective in treating angina that occurs with exertion (like beta blockers), but also angina due to spasm of the coronary arteries (like nitroglycerin). The name comes from their action of inhibiting calcium flow in micro channels in the muscular walls of the arteries as well as in the heart muscle. When these calcium channels are inhibited, the muscular wall of the arteries relaxes, the artery dilates and allows more blood flow to occur. When it occurs in the arteries of the arms and legs, blood pressure is lowered. When it occurs in the coronary arteries, angina is reduced or prevented. When it occurs in the heart muscle, the contraction force is reduced; the work of the heart is reduced. Some affect the nerve cells to the heart and may slow the heart rate. Veins also dilate, reducing the return flow of blood to the heart and also reducing the work load of the heart. The calcium that is blocked by these drugs is at a micro cellular level and has nothing to do with the calcium you may take as a supplement.

Types of Calcium Channel Blockers

The three different classes of calcium channel blockers essentially differ in their ability to dilate blood vessels, slow the heart rate and decrease the force of contraction of the heart muscle.

• Verapamil: This drug has the greatest ability to slow the heart rate and thus is also the most effective for abnormal heart rhythms. It decreases the force of contraction of the heart and is very effective for angina that occurs with exertion. It can be taken once per day and also comes in a bedtime delayed release formula for those with angina on awakening in the morning. It also causes the most constipation and the least leg swelling. It needs to be used cautiously, if at all, with beta blockers due to the heart rate lowering effects of both drugs.

• Diltiazem: This drug has an in-between ability to slow the heart rate, decrease the force of contraction of the heart muscle and dilate blood vessels. It is also effective for angina and abnormal heart rhythms. Leg swelling is potentially slightly more than with verapamil; constipation is potentially slightly less.

• Dihydropyridines: This is the largest class of calcium channel blockers. They have virtually no effect on slowing the heart rate and are therefore less effective than verapamil, diltiazem or beta blockers in treating angina. They slightly decrease the force of contraction of the heart muscle, but they are very effective blood vessel dilators. Because they are potent dilators, leg swelling is a prominent side effect, as well as dizziness, flushing and headache. Drugs in this class are nifedipine, nitrendipine, nicardipine, felodipine and amlodipine.

Side effects

The side effects vary depending on the compound as mentioned above. Leg swelling is probably the most prominent. The compounds are a very effective adjunct in the treatment of angina, especially if beta blockers cannot be tolerated.

4. Ranexa: ranolazine extended-release tablets

This is a new and unique class of drug used to reduce the frequency of angina episodes and improve exercise time before the onset of angina. Slightly less effective in women than men. Constipation is one of the more common side effects.

Putting It All Together

Most patients with chronic angina (depending of course on age and other medical problems) have had a coronary angiogram by a cardiologist and a decision was made not to do coronary bypass surgery or a stent. Treatment then usually starts with a beta blocker, aspirin, cholesterol lowering drugs and nitroglycerin sublingual (as needed). The beta blockers are gradually increased if angina occurs with most normal activities, then long acting nitroglycerin compounds are added and calcium channel blockers, if necessary. Ranexa can be added to beta blockers, nitrates and calcium channel blockers (except for diltiazem) if needed. Weight loss, aerobic exercise, and good control of blood pressure and diabetes is essential.

If angina persists at an unacceptable level, External Counterpulsation (ECP), described in the next section, is a very effective treatment. Also, reconsideration of possible bypass surgery or stents would be indicated.

Non-invasive Treatment for Angina: External Counterpulsation (ECP)

> **Fast Fact**
>
> ECP is non-invasive. It is effective in relieving angina in over 80% of the patients who are not suitable for intra-coronary stents or coronary bypass.

Mary had her first coronary bypass surgery at the age of 46. After her surgery, she gave up smoking, lost 20 pounds, adhered to a reasonable and consistent exercise program and religiously took her cholesterol lowering medications. Her routine exercise program consisted of strength training and 40 minutes of aerobic exercise on a treadmill four times per week. Almost six years after her surgery, she noticed a familiar burning sensation in her chest while on her treadmill. It was characteristic of the "indigestion" sensation she had prior to surgery.

Mary wasted little time in seeing us for these new symptoms. We performed a nuclear stress test which showed decreased blood flow to the front wall of the heart. An invasive coronary angiogram showed that three of her bypass grafts were working perfectly. The fourth graft to the branch artery in the front, called the diagonal artery, was now totally closed. It was not reachable with stents or PTCA. Her options were a repeat bypass surgery, which was not reasonable in view of the fact that she had three functioning grafts. She was entered into our ECP program. By the third week she was again symptom free. She completed her 35 visits.

A repeat nuclear stress test was normal only two months after completing ECP. Now, five years after completing ECP, she remains symptom free, her nuclear stress tests remain normal, showing normal blood flow to all walls of the heart and she continues with a normal and vigorous lifestyle.

ECP is a relatively new, noninvasive technique for providing relief to patients with chronic angina. The treatment was approved by the FDA in 1999 and is reserved for patients who continue to have angina despite medications but are not candidates for coronary bypass surgery or intra-coronary stents or PTCA.

Patients who undergo therapy with ECP may get total or partial relief from their chest pain, a reduction in the need for anti-anginal medications, and improvement in their exercise capacity and quality of life. Unlike bypass surgery and angioplasty, ECP is noninvasive, carries little risk, is relatively comfortable and requires less financial outlay than bypass or angioplasty.

ECP is administered by placing inflatable cuffs around the legs and buttocks while a patient lies comfortably on a bed. The cuffs then inflate sequentially, triggered by an electrical signal from an ECG. ECP substantially increases the blood flow to the heart and coronary arteries by pumping blood back to the coronary arteries during the resting cycle of the heart, referred to as *diastole*. Then when the heart starts to contract, referred to as the *systolic* cycle of the heart, the cuffs sequentially deflate so the heart can more easily eject blood into the aorta and major arteries of the body, essentially unloading or reducing the work on the heart.

Other organs and muscles receive their bloodflow during the systolic (contractile) phase of the cardiac cycle. The heart muscle and the coronary arteries are unique in that their blood flow occurs during the diastolic (relaxation) phase of the cardiac cycle. This makes sense, as it would be hard to push oxygenated blood into the tensely contracted heart muscle during systole. In diastole, the heart muscle is relaxed and can more easily receive blood flow.

ECP is an outpatient treatment administered for one to two hours per day for a total of 35 hours over a four to seven week period. The patient can continue his or her normal daily activities while entered in the treatment program.

Eighty percent of patients get symptomatic improvement, i.e., less angina, less shortness of breath, less use of medications, improved exercise tolerance, improved quality of life. There is also an improvement in the heart function (ejection fraction). Research data provided by us at the Orange County Heart Institute and other centers showing this improvement in heart function with ECP has led to the FDA approving ECP for congestive heart failure in 2004.

Of those patients who do improve, benefits are sustained in eighty percent of the responders at three years. Some ancillary benefits a a decrease in leg cramps, improved diabetic control, and in some men, improvement in erectile dysfunction.

The cost of a 35-hour course of ECP is significantly less expensive than angioplasty and bypass surgery. By reducing angina symptoms, it may also decrease the cost of medications, prevent hospital admissions for angina and congestive heart failure and decrease frequency of office visits to the doctor.

The history of ECP goes back to the early 1960s when published experimental work revealed the potential benefits of counterpulsation for treating CAD. There was evidence that ECP stimulated collateral coronary artery development. Collateral arteries are very small blood vessels that grow on the surface of the heart from an open coronary artery to another artery that is totally or partially blocked. It is believed that the increased pressure in the coronary artery caused by the pumping action of ECP, causes the release of a growth factor at the end of the open artery. Called *vascular endothelial growth factor (VEGF)*, it stimulates the growth of these tiny collateral arteries. Once the collaterals develop, they tend to persist until the open artery develops its own narrowing or blockage.

VEGF is a naturally occurring protein that stimulates new vessel growth which may serve as collaterals or new pathways for blood to bypass previously occluded segments. This often occurs spontaneously in the human heart. ECP accelerates and stimulates this process. It seems that an individual's capacity to develop collaterals is genetically determined. Some patients readily develop large collateral arteries relatively quickly while others develop few if any collaterals.

Our experience with ECP at the Orange County Heart Institute started in the year 2000. Since then we have successfully treated many hundreds of patients. Over 95% of them had prior coronary bypass surgery or prior intra-coronary stents. They all had changes to the coronary arteries that made them unsuitable for stents or bypass surgery. Over 90% of our patients have a significant improvement in their angina symptoms, and the vast majority are symptom free and return to normal lives. The quality of life for almost all of our patients improves dramatically. External counterpulsation is now an integral part of our cardiology practice.

5

Surgery, Stents and Lasers for Coronary Artery Disease

The surgical (invasive) treatment of coronary artery disease is similar in men and women. However, the success rates of all corrective procedures are slightly different in women compared to men. The reason for this disparity is not entirely clear.

Part of the disparity is because women develop coronary disease at an older age than men do, and surgery of this kind has a higher failure rate with advancing age. In addition, in general, the coronary arteries tend to be of smaller diameter in women than in men. The smaller the diameter of the coronary artery, the less likely a coronary bypass graft will remain open since the blood flow through the graft is slower and perhaps more likely to clot off. The smaller the diameter of the artery, the more likely scar tissue will grow and close off a small stent compared to a large diameter stent, which would need a larger amount of scar tissue to close it off.

Angioplasty (PTCA)

Angioplasty, otherwise referred to as PTCA (percutaneous transluminal coronary angioplasty), evolved in the late 1970s. Radiologists first performed balloon dilatation of atherosclerotic blockages in arteries in the legs. A Swiss radiologist, Dr. Andreas Gruntzig, performed the first angioplasty in a coronary artery in 1977. Drs. Simon Sterzer and Richard Mylar then performed this technique for the first time in the United States in 1978.

The PTCA procedure gained rapid and widespread acceptance as an alternative to coronary artery bypass graft surgery (CABG). By the early 1980s, the number of PTCA cases performed annually in the U.S. approached that of CABG surgery, and by the mid and late 1980s far outstripped the number of surgeries performed.

From the beginning, there were two problems with PTCA. The first was that of acute closure of the just opened artery. The process of opening a coronary blockage requires that hard, atherosclerotic plaque be pressed and squeezed with a rigid balloon using pressures greater than 100 pounds per square inch. This often causes a tear (dissection) within the arterial wall where the plaque has separated from the normal, non-diseased wall. Such a tear can dissect down the length of the artery and promote clot or thrombus formation, thus threatening blood flow through the artery.

This acute tear-and-clot formation could lead to a heart attack. In the early days of PTCA, a cardiac surgeon often stood by in case of an acute closure and if this occurred, the patient was rushed to the operating room for emergency CABG surgery.

These coronary dissections caused a procedural death rate of about one to three percent, and a heart attack incidence of two to four percent.

The second problem with early angioplasty was recurrence of the blockage (restenosis). Restenosis is caused by growth of scar tissue on the inner lining of the artery. In other words, a buildup of scar tissue occurs in reaction to the trauma of the high-pressure balloon dilation. Such restenosis occurred in 30 to 50 percent of the cases and was serious enough to cause a recurrence of symptoms requiring a second or third angioplasty attempt in 20 to 30 percent of the cases. Generally, such restenosis occurred within six months of the initial procedure. If recurrence did not occur within six months, that coronary lesion was generally a long-term cure.

Still, PTCA angioplasty was a very attractive alternative to CABG surgery. With PTCA, a patient's hospital stay may be one to two days and return to work in a week. CABG surgery requires a week in the hospital and several months before returning to work.

But the Achilles heel of PTCA was the restenosis in one-third of the cases. We conducted intense research for years to find a resolution to the problem. Multiple changes in technique were attempted: using a larger balloon, a smaller balloon, more pressure, less pressure, inflation for seconds, inflation for minutes—all were tried. In addition, we employed multiple medications in a futile attempt to reduce the scar formation of tissue that caused the recurrent blockage.

We tried various "niche" devices as well, with the hope that they would decrease the restenosis rate. Directional atherectomy (DCA), intracoronary lasers, rotational atherectomy, and cutting balloon angioplasty are all effective in removing plaque and opening the artery, but each of these devices have a higher retenosis rate than stents. These devices are still used in certain unique circumstances determined by the cardiologist.

Stents

The greatest success in the historical development of percutaneous coronary intervention—this means fixing the coronary artery through a catheter-based procedure like PTCA, stents, lasers, etc.—came with the release of intracoronary stents, which are metal coils implanted in the artery after balloon inflation.

By the early-to-mid-1990s, stents became effective and widely used, greatly improving the two greatest challenges to PTCA. First, stents are able to tack up and stabilize any dissection that occurs when the balloon is inflated. This has greatly reduced the need for emergency CABG surgery and decreased the incidence of heart attack following PTCA. Of greater benefit is a significant of drop in deaths due to PTCA. Where previous mortality rates were one to three percent, most institutions now have death rates of less than 0.5 percent.

Second, stents have reduced restenosis rates from 20 to 30%

to as low as five to ten percent.

Currently, nearly one million PTCA procedures and half a million surgical CABGs are performed annually in the United States.

Rarely, stents will cause a clot when first placed. This occurs less than one percent of the time. The best prevention is to take a combination of aspirin and Ticlid or Plavix. These three medications are inhibitors of platelets, the components in blood that initiate the clotting process. Ideally, Ticlid and Plavix should be taken immediately after stent placement, and then taken afterwards for two to four weeks for bare metal stents, and for over a year for drug coated stents.

Stents are placed at the same time that balloon angioplasty is performed. First, we dilate the coronary artery with a balloon. Then, while the artery is wide open, we remove the balloon and insert the stent. The stent comes mounted or crimped on a deflated balloon. It is positioned in the correct location within the coronary artery; the balloon upon which the stent is mounted is then inflated. The stent expands to its open position and remains imbedded against the coronary wall. We then deflate the delivery balloon and remove it. The stent remains imbedded in the artery wall.

Usually a patient is in the hospital for twenty-four hours following stent placement. Potential complications include a one percent chance of heart attack, emergency surgery, stroke, or femoral artery hemorrhage.

Recently, coated stents have been developed. These are similar in design to the traditional "bare metal" stent, except a drug is imbedded in the wire struts of the stent. The drug is slowly released into the wall of the artery when the stent is expanded. The drug inhibits formation of scar tissue, thus reducing the restenosis rate to around two to five percent.

Stents are a dramatic advance in the treatment of coronary disease. The restenosis rate after stenting is higher if the artery is small in diameter (2.5mm), or narrowed with a long (20mm) segment of plaque. Now these smaller arteries and longer blockages can be treated with coated stents with an acceptable restenosis rate.

Early reports suggested there were more clots and deaths with the coated stents compared to bare metal stents. It turns out that there is less danger with the coated stents as long as Plavix is used for at least 12 months or more. Dissolvable stents are under investigation. They will scaffold the artery for the first six months while the artery heals. The stent will then dissolve and leave a natural lining in the artery making it less prone to clot formation compared to metal stents (even though with metal stents the risk of clotting is still very small). Whether dissolvable stents will offer any short or long term benefit over present bare metal and coated stents remains to be seen.

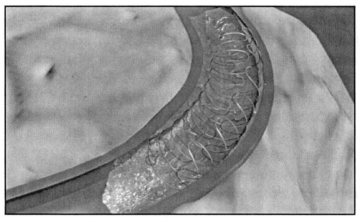

Stent expanded in coronary artery

Recent reports suggested that medical treatment is just as effective as angioplasty in treating angina and preventing death, except for heart attacks, in which case angioplasty is superior. However, the data was collected before the era of coated stents. The bottom line: when coated stents are used to treat a severe narrowing in a coronary artery which supplies blood flow to a large amount of heart muscle, they are superior to medications in treating angina and protecting the heart from damage.

In-stent Restenosis

Coronary stenting has established itself as an effective procedure for the treatment of coronary artery disease. Stents have significantly reduced the incidence of restenosis. Restenosis with plain balloon angioplasty can be as high as 30 to 40%. With the use of stents, this problem of recurrent blockage is most often reduced to 5 to 15%.

However, when restenosis does occur within the coronary stent, it can be extremely difficult to treat. Once this scarring occurs within a stent, there is a high rate of recurrence after treatment. Restenosis within the stent appears on an angiogram as a discrete, focal lesion or as diffuse thickening of the inner lining of the artery.

Treatment strategies for in-stent restenosis include mechanical compression of the in-stent scar tissue with balloon angioplasty. This involves simply placing a balloon within the stent and inflating it to a high pressure, thereby compressing the recurrent plaque. A unique type of balloon has small razor blades that expand and slice the scar tissue and is more effective than plain balloon angioplasty. These new balloons are called *cutting balloons.* Another more effective technique is to clean out the scar tissue with a cutting balloon, then place a new coated stent within the old one: a so-called "stent sandwich."

Another treatment option involves dissolving the scar tissue either with the excimer laser (ELCA) or with a rotating burr (rotational atherectomy), or with radiation therapy (brachytherapy). This involves passing some form of radioactive beads into the stent for a brief exposure of the scar tissue to the source of radiation. Such exposure appears to prevent the scar tissue from recurring. The type of treatment depends on the choice of the cardiologists, however, brachytherapy is used less often than the more effective and easier "stent sandwich."

Atherectomy

Atherectomy catheters, which actually remove plaque from the artery wall, were the next device development after balloon angioplasty. We called the removal of plaque using these devices atherectomy (excision of atheroma). These devices took on several forms. The first to gain FDA approval was the directional

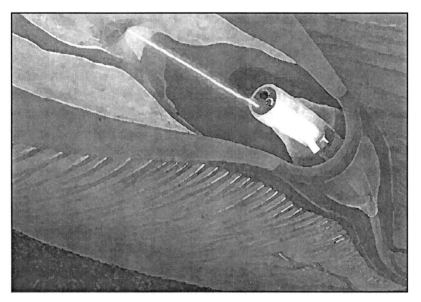

Excimer laser vaporizing plaque

coronary atherectomy (DCA). This device actually cut and re-moved the atherosclerotic tissue. Doctors embraced it with much enthusiasm. However, studies failed to show any successful re-duction in restenosis rates compared to PTCA. DCA is still very effective at removing plaque in the mouth (ostium) of an artery or at a branch point (bifurcation).

Laser Atherectomy

After DCA came laser atherectomy. There was much excite-ment around laser development. Institutions spent years of re-search and millions of dollars identifying the right wavelength of laser energy and perfecting a catheter that could deliver the laser inside the coronary artery. The current laser most commonly used is the excimer laser, referred to as a "cold" laser because it does not induce burning and chafing of the tissue.

In comparative studies with angioplasty, the current excimer laser system (manufactured by Spectranetics) again revealed no improvement in preventing restenosis. However, there may exist several potential roles for the excimer laser. One is using a laser wire that can cross totally blocked coronary arteries. A second

89

use would be debulking plaque prior to placing a stent. This debulking or vaporization of plaque may reduce the chance of restenosis.

A third use of the excimer laser might be treatment of ostial lesions, blockages that exist where the coronary artery arises from the aorta. These blockages are very resistant to angioplasty because the muscular aorta tends to recoil after balloon dilation. Vaporizing the fibrous and muscular tissue at the mouth of these coronary arteries may be more effective in preventing recurrence.

Rotoblator Atherectomy

The third generation of atherectomy, rotoblator atherectomy, uses a tiny, football shaped burr coated with diamond fragments that spins at 150,000 to 200,000 rpm. This amazing engineering feat allows for the effective obliteration of hard plaque in heavily calcified arteries. Again, restenosis rates are not greatly improved. However, rotoblator atherectomy is very effective at treating hard, calcified arteries in diabetics and in older patients.

Surgical Intervention and Therapy

Coronary Artery Bypass Graft (CABG) Surgery

Surgeons first performed coronary artery bypass graft surgery thirty years ago in the treatment of coronary arteries occluded with atherosclerotic plaque. It is a successful surgical technique, well refined and studied. Patients undergoing CABG surgery have coronary artery disease that is not amenable to balloon angioplasty for the following reasons.

If the artery is totally occluded, sometimes the guide wire cannot be passed and therefore a balloon or stent cannot be placed in the artery. CABG surgery is currently the only way to effectively re-establish arterial blood flow beyond the total blockage. In addition, blockages may be so numerous and extensive that angioplasty would not be as effective as bypass.

Involvement of the left main coronary artery, the main artery supplying blood flow to the entire left side of the heart, is best treated with CABG since any complication could jeopardize coronary blood flow to a large area of heart muscle. This could result in death or severe complications, although there are certain rare situations where stenting of the left main coronary is performed.

A cardiothoracic surgeon performs CABG surgery. The operative procedure takes two to four hours or more. Three to seven days of postoperative stay in the hospital are required. Traditional CABG surgery, done through a midline incision in the breastbone (sternum), requires six to ten weeks of recovery time before the patient can resume all physical activities. This delay is required for healing of the breastbone.

Complications of CABG surgery are those of any major surgery: infection, kidney failure, stroke or death. Death rates are dependent on the risk evaluation of the patient before surgery. Factors that increase the likelihood of death or some complication include age, female sex, diabetes, cigarette smoking, renal insufficiency or failure, obesity, and prior myocardial infarction with poor left-heart function. A good surgical program has a mortality rate of one to five percent. As lower-risk patients are successfully treated with PTCA and stents, the complexity of CABG patients and their risks increase. The low surgical-mortality rate of previous years may rise as patient complexity increases.

Problems with Bypass Grafts-Veins

The greatest challenge to successful CABG surgery has been late closure of bypass grafts. Initially, veins were taken from the leg and used as conduits for the bypass. One end of a vein segment was attached to the aorta, while the far end was attached to the coronary artery beyond the blockage. These vein grafts can occlude shortly after surgery if a clot forms within the graft or if the graft closes due to inflammation. Fortunately, this is unusual and can be prevented by taking aspirin postoperatively.

Late closure of grafts can also occur years later. Studies have shown that after ten years up to 50% of grafts may be closed. It is common for some patients to have undergone surgery two or three times. With each subsequent surgery, the complication rate gets higher, and it becomes more and more difficult for the surgeon to find adequate bypass-graft conduits. Grafts in subsequent surgeries do not last as long.

Once a bypass graft is inserted, the disease in the native coronary artery often progresses to total occlusion. This goes unnoticed by the patient since adequate blood flow is delivered beyond the occlusion via the newly placed graft. If the graft then closes years later, the patient will have no adequate blood flow. A heart attack can occur, or if the patient has developed collateral blood flow from other arteries, she may develop chronic recurrent angina.

Arterial Bypass Grafts

Grafts are veins taken from the legs or from arteries along the inner rib cage called internal mammary arteries, or arteries from the forearm, called radial arteries and on rare occasions, the arteries that supply the upper portion of the stomach, called gastro epiploic arteries. To reduce the incidence of *vein* bypass grafts, *arterial* grafts are now widely used. Initially, the internal mammary artery (IMA) was the principal alternative to vein grafts. The internal mammary artery comes off the subclavian artery under the collarbone. It runs on the underside of the rib cage to supply blood flow to the chest wall. Fortunately, there is a second, duplicate flow of blood to this same region from alternative arteries. The heart surgeon leaves the IMA attached to its source on the subclavian artery and redirects the distal end to an attachment site on the diseased coronary artery. These arterial grafts have a long-term patency, that is, they remain open at a rate of 95% after ten years. Vein grafts at ten years have a 30% patency rate, that is, about 65 to 70% of vein grafts are closed ten years after surgery. Grafts from cadavers are rarely used since they have a very low long-term patency rate.

Bypass Graft Sources

There are two IMAs, right and left. If both are used, there is a possible compromise of the arterial flow to the incised sternum. This can lead to a higher rate of poor bone sealing and infection. For this reason, some surgeons will only use one IMA. Second, the IMA cannot reach all portions of the coronary arte-

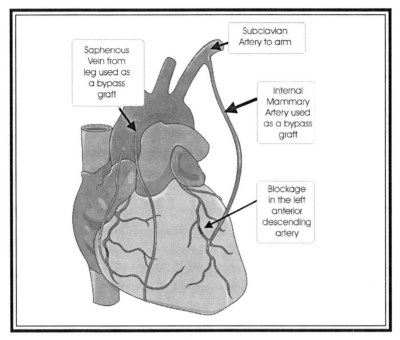

Saphenous Vein from leg used as a bypass graft

Subclavian Artery to arm

Internal Mammary Artery used as a bypass graft

Blockage in the left anterior descending artery

Heart With Bypass Grafts

rial tree, thus limiting its use for some bypass sites. In these cases, the surgeon has three options: use a vein graft (with the knowledge that it is less likely to survive a lifetime), use the gastroepiploic artery or use a "free" arterial graft.

Free arterial grafts come from an artery somewhere else in the body, usually a radial artery taken from the wrist. Arteries do not have as much alternative, or backup, flow as do veins, so a radial artery segment can only be taken if the hand has adequate blood flow from the ulnar artery, a second artery in the wrist supplying blood flow to the hand.

The surgeon can detach the gastroepiploic artery and redirect its flow to the undersurface of the heart. As with the internal mammary arteries, the gastroepiploic artery is limited in its ability to reach far enough when inserted onto the heart. Complications include decreased blood flow to the stomach that can cause indigestion or ulcers.

Bypass Surgery Or PTCA?

Many studies predate the current use of modern stents that greatly reduce the complications of PTCA and restenosis problems. In these studies, CABG surgery looks very favorable in patients with multiple lesions greater than or equal to three, and especially in patients with diabetes who are prone to extensive disease and higher rates of restenosis following PTCA. However, multi-vessel drug coated stents compare favorably to multiple vessel CABG, especially for younger patients with multi-vessel disease.

The problem with performing CABG surgery in a young patient is that eventual graft occlusion leaves the patient no alternative other than repeat bypass surgery. If a 40-year-old patient undergoes CABG surgery, he may then develop symptoms of new disease or occluded bypass grafts. A second surgery may be performed at age 50, a third at age 60. Sometimes the interval between surgeries is much shorter. Each subsequent surgery becomes more difficult. PTCA may then not be an alternative because the native coronary artery has probably progressed to uncrossable (with a wire) occlusion.

In comparison, if a young patient undergoes multi-vessel PTCA, the native arteries remain open. If recurrent symptoms occur, or if new occlusions are detected by stress testing, a wire can be passed and a repeat PTCA performed with a stent placed. Over a long period of time, many more options are available to the patient if the native artery remains patent.

It is now becoming apparent that multiple arteries can be treated with coated stents with comparable results to multiple vessel coronary bypass surgery. Diabetics and those with smaller coronary arteries, however, still seem to do better with coronary bypass versus coated stents if multiple arteries need to be fixed.

New Surgical Techniques
Off-Pump or Beating Heart Bypass Surgery

Of all the recent developments in surgical technique, off-pump bypass leads to shorter hospitalizations, less blood loss, quicker recovery and lower complication rates. This technique involves opening the sternum in the same manner as traditional bypass surgery. However, instead of stopping the heart from beating and placing the patient on the heart-lung bypass pump while the grafts are sewn onto the heart, the heart is allowed to keep beating while the grafts are sewn on. To sew the grafts onto the beating heart, a device called an Octopus has been developed to hold still the section of the coronary artery being bypassed. As a rule, the front coronary arteries are more suited to this technique. It must also be the patient's first surgery, that is, it can't be a redo CABG.

Minimally Invasive Heart Surgery

New developments in bypass surgery include the evolution of "minimally invasive" surgery using Heart Port TM technology, in which we place a patient on a heart-lung bypass machine without the chest and sternum fully opened. A limited incision can be made in the chest wall through which the surgeon performs the CABG surgery.

Using complex catheters placed on the venous and arterial sides of the heart through various puncture or entry sites, the surgeon stops the patient's heart, maintaining brain and body blood flow with a heart-lung bypass machine. With the heart "stopped," the surgeon can replace a valve or insert a bypass graft. This technology has moderate success and has not gained widespread use.

Trans-Myocardial Laser Revascularization (TMLR)

This is one of the latest developments in cardiac surgery. In this procedure, the laser pierces the surface of the heart muscle, creating small channels. These channels allow for blood from within the ventricle to percolate up into the heart muscle, supplying oxygenated blood.

Some call the procedure "lizard surgery." Lizards and other reptiles do not have coronary arteries to supply blood to the heart muscle which is Swiss-cheese-like in appearance. The reptilian heart muscle receives its oxygenated blood via percolation of oxygenated blood from the main pumping chamber up through

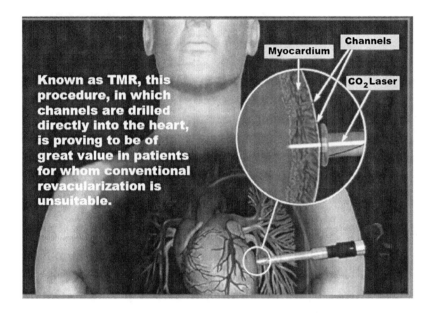

Known as TMR, this procedure, in which channels are drilled directly into the heart, is proving to be of great value in patients for whom conventional revacularization is unsuitable.

Myocardium

Channels

CO_2 Laser

the "holes" into the muscle.

It is a technique used in heart patients to recreate blood flow to diseased heart muscle where no other alternative exists. Some patients have an occluded coronary artery, thus preventing the performance of PTCA; they also have no vessel acceptable to receive a bypass graft. If the surgeon can see no vessel big enough to graft following angiography, it is very unlikely that an acceptable vessel will be found once the chest is opened and the heart exposed. In these patients, TMLR may provide an alternative way of recreating blood flow.

This procedure currently can only be performed by placing the laser on the outside surface of the heart where it blasts a small channel though the heart muscle (myocardium). Surprisingly, the heart does not bleed out, as one would expect when multiple holes are created. The squeezing of the heart causes the surface channels to close spontaneously via thrombosis. The laser-created channels, however, do remain open on the inner lining of the heart muscle (endocardium). Hence, to get adequate exposure to allow the laser to be positioned, surgery must be performed either via a full sternotomy where the breastbone is split and separated, exposing the heart, or via a limited incision between the ribs, as is done with minimally invasive surgery.

Research and development are now exploring a technique in which TMLR can be done via a catheter placed within the left ventricle coming up from a puncture site in the femoral artery, similar to the performance of PTCA.

Gene therapy and stem cell therapy

Both therapies are still investigational and early results are mixed. Basically they involve injecting a substance into the coronary artery that supplies insufficient blood to the heart muscle due to severe blockages in the coronary arteries. In general, these patients have angina and are not candidates for stents, lasers or bypass surgery.

The injected gene or stem cell is supposed to evolve into new arteries to supply blood to the heart muscle, and therefore relieve angina.

In summary, surgical therapy for coronary artery disease is rapidly changing. The amazing benefits of coated stents have enabled cardiologists to safely cut down on the number of patients who need to go to coronary bypass surgery. A shorter hospital stay, quicker return to work, and a rapid resumption of normal lifestyle, as well as lower hospital costs, are all benefits of the modern coated-stent era.

6

Shortness of Breath and Congestive Heart Failure

K N is a 36-year-old woman who had been having cough and chest congestion for two weeks during which time she noticed a weight gain of 12 pounds. When she finally came to the hospital she was diagnosed with congestive heart failure.

What is congestive heart failure?

Congestive heart failure, (CHF) often called simply "heart failure," sounds scary, as if your heart could stop and death strike at any moment. It's not all that gloomy. Millions of people live with heart failure and with proper care, conduct relatively normal lives. Usually heart failure develops over a period of time as a result of an underlying problem such as coronary artery disease, high blood pressure, or heart valve or muscle defects. The same risk factors for coronary artery disease are involved in heart failure.

CHF is not a disease; it's a condition or a process in which the heart is unable to pump enough blood forward to meet the needs of the body's tissues. Don't get the wrong idea. The heart doesn't "fail" in that it stops beating, as it does with a severe heart attack. Instead, it weakens, usually over the course of months or years, resulting in poor blood pumping ability. Remember that the heart is basically a pump to deliver oxygen-rich blood to all parts of the body for vital energy. In people with heart failure, this ability has been weakened resulting in a back-up of fluid in the lungs and other tissues. Patients will then have shortness of breath, fatigue and swelling. Everyday activities such as walking, climbing stairs, and doing chores around the house, can become difficult.

Heart failure can occur at any age, however, it is more common in older people. As the older population keeps growing over the next decades, we expect to see more people living with heart failure. At this time, about five million Americans live with CHF.

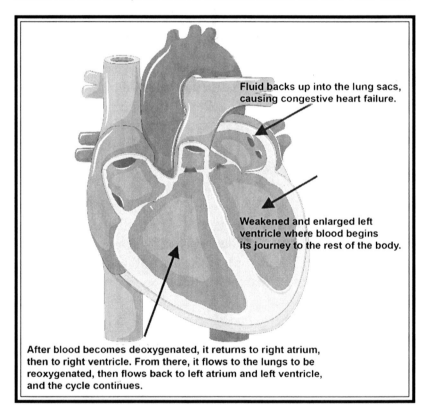

Fluid backs up into the lung sacs, causing congestive heart failure.

Weakened and enlarged left ventricle where blood begins its journey to the rest of the body.

After blood becomes deoxygenated, it returns to right atrium, then to right ventricle. From there, it flows to the lungs to be reoxygenated, then flows back to left atrium and left ventricle, and the cycle continues.

To understand what causes CHF, it will help to understand how the heart functions and propels blood throughout the body. (See illustration.)

The heart has two sides and each side has two chambers. The top chamber is called the atrium and the bottom chamber is called the ventricle. Usually, the blood is pumped from the left ventricle, the bottom left chamber, to the rest of the body. This blood is oxygenated and full of nutrients for the different organs. As the blood travels throughout the body, it eventually loses its oxygen and empties into the right atrium, the top right chamber of the heart. This blood then goes downward into the right ventricle, the bottom right chamber, where it is sent to the lungs. It is there that the exchange of oxygen occurs, and the blood becomes oxygenated. As it leaves the lungs, the blood flows into the left atrium, the top left chamber of the heart and from there into the left ventricle and the cycle will continue. Now, either side of the heart can be involved in heart failure. That is why we see different symptoms in different patients. However, it is usually the left side that loses its ability to pump efficiently and, as a consequence of this change, the right side follows.

When the left side starts failing, the left ventricle is most affected. This is called left-sided heart failure or left ventricular heart failure. The left ventricle is a strong chamber since it pumps blood to the rest of the body. If it weakens, it will affect the overall function of the heart and what we refer to as the ejection fraction (EF) of the heart. It is important for patients with heart failure to know this number. (See Chapter One for a full description of EF.) The physician, upon suspecting heart failure, will usually order an echocardiogram, an ultrasound of the heart, to assess the functions of both sides of the heart and to assess the ejection fraction of the heart.

Symptoms and diagnosis

When the left side of the heart fails, the blood that was supposed to go forward will back up into the lungs and fluid can leak into the lungs. This will cause shortness of breath (dyspnea), inability to walk and perform chores, and waking up in the middle of the night. The patient will need more pillows to sleep at night. It can also cause coughing at night (nocturnal cough).

The medical term for this fluid "back up" is pulmonary edema. As the heart failure worsens and the pump becomes weaker, the flow of blood will slow down and eventually other tissues in the body can experience leaking of the fluid, called edema. Eventually this inability to pump the blood forward can cause the patient to feel tired and anxious. Patients with severe heart failure do not have a good appetite and become very thin. This all happens as the body adjusts itself to receiving less blood. Blood will be shifted away from the muscles, causing fatigue, and from the digestive system, resulting in lack of appetite and feeling full, and into the vital organs, the heart and the brain.

When the right side of the heart fails, right ventricular heart failure, it is usually a result of previous left-sided failure. The blood then backs up in the veins, the vessels that bring the blood from all the tissues *back* to the heart. This back-up results in swelling of the lower extremities, the legs and the ankles. It can also be seen as enlargment of the liver, since the liver is the last stop before the blood flows back into the right side of the heart. Patients may also have more prominent neck veins.

How can you recognize symptoms?

1. Cough
Cough at any time, but usually at night, can be one of the first symptoms of heart failure. It usually is associated with white-pink mucus. Not all coughs mean that you have heart failure. They can also come from stomach problems, lung ailments or medications (most notably ACE inhibitor medications like Lisinopril).

2. Shortness of breath
With activity or at rest. When it happens at rest, it usually signifies that the heart failure is advanced. You may also experience difficulty lying flat or waking in the middle of night feeling short of breath. As with cough, shortness of breath does not always mean you have heart failure. Lung problems, lack of exercise, obesity and even kidney disease can cause shortness of breath.

3. Fatigue

As we explained before, fatigue will eventually occur as the heart cannot withstand the demands of the body and the muscles may not receive enough blood. But fatigue can also result from deconditioning and lack of exercise.

4. Edema

The buildup of fluid in different tissues will happen over time. Since heart failure is a slow process at the beginning, patients may not notice subtle changes. Edema in the legs may or may not be a sign of heart failure. If the veins in the legs become incompetent to send the blood back to the heart, then there will be leaking of fluid into the tissues and consequently leg swelling. Leg edema can also result from kidney diseases. A patient may also complain about swelling in her abdomen, or the physician may feel an enlarged liver on physical exam.

Common tests used in diagnosing and managing CHF

1. Blood tests

Heart failure patients may find themselves in the laboratory many times a year. This happens because they are usually on large quantities of medications that can interact with each other and can increase or decrease vital electrolytes in the blood. Physicians follow the change in the electrolytes closely.

Another reason why patients may have their blood tested is to determine the level of the hormone B-type natriuretic peptide (BNP). Currently, emergency departments use the results of the BNP level to assist them in deciding whose shortness of breath is secondary to heart failure and whose is not. This easy to perform blood test is also available in the outpatient laboratory. Elevated levels of BNP are seen when the heart is damaged and is in failure. This hormone is actually secreted to help with excretion of the extra fluid in the body as a result of heart failure. As an outpatient tool, its level assists the physician to monitor the patient and it can help predict the prognosis in patients with heart disease and heart failure. Frequent measurement of potassium levels and measurements of kidney function (serum creatinine) are needed since the use of large amounts of diuretics to reduce fluids will affect potassium levels and sometimes kidney function.

2. Chest X-Ray

In addition to blood tests, patients will have chest x-rays (CXR) on occasion, especially at the time of their first visit, to aid the physician in assessing congestion in the lungs and the size of the heart.

3. Echocardiography

Ultrasonography of the heart is called echocardiography. Using this non-invasive device, the physician can see the patient's heart structures, the movements of the heart muscle, the ejection fraction of the heart, and the presence of tightness or leakage of the heart valves. It is important to know whether the ejection fraction of the heart is normal or reduced since it can help in assessing the cause of the heart failure. It is highly recommended for patients with heart failure to know their ejection fraction and its trend.

4. ECG

The ECG does not diagnose heart failure, but it is an important management tool. The ECG may reveal evidence of an old heart attack, an abnormal heart rhythm, or an unusually slow heart rate, all of which may contribute to the deterioration of heart function.

What are the causes of CHF?

1. Coronary artery disease

When there is disease in the arteries that feed the heart, less blood reaches the heart muscle. This can result in injury to the heart muscle. While this occurs, the healthy part has to work harder, which can lead to heart failure. The unhealthy muscle can also be "dead" as a result of a heart attack. This leaves the healthy part to pump and work harder. If the patient's primary cause of heart failure is coronary heart disease, she may benefit from a heart catheterization to assess the anatomy of the heart vessels. Some patients' symptoms improve after bypass surgery or angioplasty.

2. High blood pressure

The risk of heart failure increases two to three times when high blood pressure is not controlled. This leads to the heart working harder and, over time, the chambers get weaker and the muscle walls thicken and stiffen. Eventually the heart muscle loses its ability to contract and relax adequately and congestive heart failure ensues. Hypertensive heart disease refers to these deleterious effects of uncontrolled hypertension on the pumping function of the heart.

3. Disease of the heart muscle (cardiomyopathy)

Viral infections, drug abuse, alcohol abuse, and inflammation of the heart muscle can result in heart failure.

Heart failure can also occur during or right after pregnancy. Although many patients recover from what is known as postpartum cardiomyopathy, they are recommended against becoming pregnant again.

4. Heart valve disease

Whether the disease of the valves is present at birth (congenital) or as a result of an infection (endocarditis), it can result in malfunctioning of the valve. The valve may not open adequately (a stenotic or narrowed heart valve) or the valve may not close properly, leading to excessive leaking of the valve (a regurgitant valve). This creates a larger work load on the heart muscle, eventually leading to heart failure.

5. Congenital heart disease

Because of an abnormality present at birth, there may be chambers or valves of the heart that do not work properly. Therefore, the healthy and normal part has to pump harder, increasing the risk for heart failure. Holes between the upper two chambers or between the lower two chambers of the heart are referred to as

ASDs (atrial septal defects) and VSDs (ventricular septal defects), respectively. These are two of the more common congenital defects easily diagnosed with an echocardiogram.

6. Diabetes

Patients with diabetes usually suffer from obesity and high blood pressure adding to their risk for heart failure. The effects of severely elevated blood sugars have a direct negative effect on the function of the heart, as well as an indirect negative effect by contributing to the risk factors that promote coronary artery disease.

7. Other causes

Lung disease, arrhythmia, severe anemia, hyperthyroidism, pregnancy and connective tissue diseases are other causes of heart failure.

How do we correct heart failure?

First of all, heart failure is usually not curable. People learn to "live" with it. First the heart starts compensating for its weakness by becoming enlarged to pump more blood. The heart rate will increase to send more blood out to the body. It can also become thicker as it tries to get stronger to pump the blood out. What the patient can do is to change her diet, add an appropriate exercise regimen and take prescribed medications.

It is important to avoid being exposed to colds and flu. Heart failure patients are more susceptible to acquiring upper respiratory infections which can worsen their heart failure. Heart failure patients should receive yearly flu vaccinations and the one-time pneumonia vaccine.

1.Diet

Appropriate caloric intake

Patients with heart disease can improve their symptoms and be more involved in their own lives and the lives of their loved ones if they adhere to a healthy diet. Obesity is a strong contributor to heart failure and loss of body fat may go a long way in improving heart function.

Sodium restriction

Sodium restriction in your diet is critical. The kidneys react to CHF by retaining sodium; this causes water retention. Sodium is excreted by taking diuretics, but the restriction of your dietary intake of sodium is equally important. For mild or moderate CHF, you should ingest less than two grams of sodium daily. For severe CHF, a patient may be restricted to less than one gram of sodium daily. In 2006, the American Medical Association recommended that healthy individuals consume only between 1,300 milligrams and 1,800 milligrams a day of sodium from all sources, the levels dependent upon physical activity. Athletes and those who work out vigorously could tolerate up to 3,000 milligrams a day. Other major health organizations such as the National Institutes of Health and American Dietetic Association have joined with the AMA in their strong recommendation.

• Excess water can make your heart work harder, elevate your blood pressure, and aggravate symptoms of congestive heart failure.
• Many canned, packaged and frozen foods are high in sodium. Reading labels can help you choose foods with lower salt content. Be aware of foods made with high salt levels, such as ham and pickles.

Fluid intake restriction

A recommendation that you should drink plenty of water does not apply to patients with heart failure. As we discussed earlier, the inability of the heart to pump the blood efficiently can result in fluid accumulation in the tissues. The class of medication called diuretics or water pills (discussed later in the chapter), can help to get rid of the excess fluid in the body. However, patients should also track fluid intake. Limit yourself to eight cups a day. This includes any type of fluid, including water and food that is liquid in consistency.

It is important for patients to weigh themselves every day, preferably in the morning wearing the same amount of clothing. Keeping track of your weight will help you and your physician determine if extra fluid is accumulating. This in turn will guide the physician in adjusting your medication and your fluid intake. About three or more pounds in one day or about five or more pounds in one week are considered sudden weight gain by most physicians.

Alcohol consumption

As we discussed earlier in the chapter, some patients may have cardiomyopathy as a result of alcoholism. These patients should never drink again. Alcohol has a negative effect on the ability of the heart to contract and will worsen heart failure.

Caffeine intake

Caffeine increases stress on the heart. It is recommended for patients with heart failure to limit the intake of caffeine and to avoid it if severe heart failure exists.

2. Exercise and stress

Exercise is recommended for its positive effect on the heart and quality of life. The important message is not to get discouraged when first starting. Exercise programs should be discussed with the physician. Cardiac rehabilitation programs help patients start slowly and increase their exercise tolerance gradually. In addition to aerobic exercise like walking, bicycling and swimming, weight and strength training are essential in managing heart failure over the long term.

Patients are also encouraged to rest every day. When you rest, you allow the heart to work at an easier pace and give it time to relax.

It is very important to learn strategies to cope with stress. The physical stress that follows an emotional stress is harmful to a failing heart.

3. Medications

Many patients with heart failure will be taking a combination of medications that have been shown to improve the function of the heart and quality of life. The following are the most commonly prescribed medications.

Diuretics (water pills)

Commonly used diuretics are Lasix (furosemide), Diuril (hydrochlorothiazide, HCTZ), Bumex, Demadex, Lozol, and Zaroxolyn.

Diuretics are prescribed when there is fluid buildup in the body. They cause an increase in urine production by removing more sodium and water from the blood. By decreasing the extra fluid, there is less work for the heart and less fluid buildup in the lungs, ankles, legs and other tissues. However, potassium loss also occurs with the loss of sodium. Potassium loss causes muscle cramping, fatigue, and cardiac arrhythmia. Potassium replacement in the form of tablets or liquid is often required. You can also replace potassium by eating bananas, cantaloupes, and drinking orange juice.

In case of sudden weight gain, the dosage of diuretics will be increased to remove the excess fluid. Some patients may be given an individual dose regimen.

The physician may use a combination of two diuretics which work at different levels in the kidney. This combination therapy is usually done for a short period of time to avoid dangerous electrolyte imbalance. Furthermore, some of the diuretics are more powerful, and patients may be switched from one to the other based on their needs.

Digoxin (Lanoxin, Digitek)

This medication has been around for over 200 years and its role in heart failure has been studied repeatedly. It comes from the plant foxglove (*digitalis purpurea*) and has been shown to cause an increase in exercise tolerance and probably a decrease in the number of hospitalizations secondary to heart failure. However, it does not affect the contractility of the heart.

Digitalis can become a toxic drug if its blood-level percentage becomes too high. Its dangerous effects are much worse in the presence of hypokalemia (low serum potassium levels). Since most patients with CHF take diuretics, and diuretics can cause hypokalemia, serum potassium and digitalis levels require periodic monitoring.

ACE Inhibitors (Angiotensin-Converting Enzyme Inhibitors)

These medicines are now the first–choice treatment for slowing the progression of heart failure. They belong to the category of drugs known as vasodilators, meaning that they cause expansion of blood vessels leading to lower blood pressure and less work for the heart. Originally, they were developed to treat high blood pressure. Commonly used ACE inhibitors include Capoten (captopril), Vasotec (enalapril), Prinivil or Zestril (lisinopril), Accupril, and many others.

One common side effect of ACE inhibitors that occurs in as many as 10 to 20% of patients, is a dry cough or tickle in the back of the throat. This resolves with discontinuation of the medicine. Patients can also develop dizziness and weakness when first starting the medication. ACE inhibitors can also increase the level of potassium in the blood, so patients may need periodic monitoring of potassium levels, especially if they are also taking different types of diuretics and potassium supplements.

Since these medications reduce blood pressure, physicians will check blood pressure regularly when these drugs are initiated. They are titrated to the lowest tolerable blood pressure. A low blood pressure is acceptable as long as there are no complaints of fatigue, dizziness or falls.

ARBs (Angiotensin II Receptor Blockers)

Losartan (Cozaar), valsartan (Diovan), irbesartan (Avapro), and candesartan (Atacand) are the drugs in this family.

These drugs usually replace the ACE inhibitors when patients complain of dry cough. They also decrease the blood pressure. They do not appear to have significant side effects, however, they have not shown any advantage over ACE inhibitors, and therefore, their use is usually second to ACE inhibitors or sometimes in combination. As in the case of ACE inhibitors, blood pressure monitoring will be done to ensure that the reduction in blood pressure is in the acceptable range. Your cardiologist may choose to start with an ARB medication over an ACE-inhibitor.

Beta Blockers (Beta-Adrenergic Blocking Agents)

Carvedilol (Coreg), metoprolol (Lopressor, Toprol XL), and atenolol belong to this category. The use of beta blockers is a newer treatment for CHF in the past decade. It seems paradoxical to use beta blockers since they block the effect of adrenaline and other potentially strong stimulants to heart function. It used to be thought that beta blockers were actually contraindicated in patients with CHF, but we have discovered that they can block deleterious neurohormonal reactions that the body inappropriately creates in reaction to CHF. These neurohormonal substances make the heart beat faster and more forcefully. By blocking these chemicals, this class of drugs reduces the heart rate, and slows the contraction of the heart, resulting in less work for the ailing organ.

The newest beta blocker approved for congestive heart failure is Coreg (carvedilol). Coreg is different from the other beta blockers, since it also has alpha blocking characteristics. With its alpha blocking capabilities, Coreg relaxes the arteries and therefore reduces the workload on the heart even further. It is used in patients with heart failure and high blood pressure. In patients with low ejection fraction, studies show that there are improvements in the overall function of the heart and eventually the EF. Patients will have scheduled echocardiograms while being treated with Coreg to assess the EF. It usually takes about six months to witness a remarkable improvement.

Beta blockers have to be taken cautiously and selectively; we start at low doses and gradually increase over time. Patients should be carefully monitored for side effects, such as heart block, low blood pressure, and low heart rate, and their other medications adjusted accordingly.

Aldosterone Blockers

The two drugs of this class on the market are Aldactone (spironolactone) and Inspra (eplerenone).

This class of drugs blocks the hormone aldosterone which acts on the kidney and causes fluid and salt retention, two factors that worsen heart failure. By blocking the hormone, these drugs work as diuretics. Patients will have loss of fluid without the loss of potassium. That is why these drugs are called "potassium-sparing" diuretics. Studies have shown that by blocking the action of this hormone, the risk of death and number of hospitalizations will be decreased.

Some of the more common side effects of these drugs are gynecomastia (breast tissue enlargement), increased hair growth in women, and an increase in plasma potassium. Physicians usually follow their patients' electrolytes regularly when the patients are taking multiple medications that can affect the potassium.

Nitrates and hydralazine

As discussed before, vasodilators expand the blood vessels which eventually results in less workload for the heart. When patients cannot tolerate ACE inhibitors, they may sometimes be placed on a combination of oral nitrates and hydralazine to improve their symptoms and tolerance for exercise. However, this combination is not a first-choice option. This combination has been used for many years by cardiologists in patients with severe heart failure who do not respond to other drug therapies. BiDil (isosorbide dinitrate/hydralizine HCI) was recently approved as a fixed-dose combination of nitrate and hydralazine for treatment of heart failure in black patients. It has been reported that black patients do not respond well to ACE-inhibitors—the first line of treatment in patients with heart failure. BiDil has been shown to reduce mortality in black patients with heart failure when added to their regimen of medications including ACE inhibitors.

Aspirin

Aspirin is in the class of the medication called NSAIDs or non-steroid anti-inflammatory drugs. It is highly recommended in men above the age of 50 for prevention and also secondary treatment of heart disease. However, in women, this drug is recommended when there are sufficient risk factors to place the person at risk for heart disease, or if the patient has coronary calcium on an EBCT heart scan. In women who do have heart disease or diabetes, aspirin is prescribed. Studies have revealed that women may suffer from stomach problems while taking aspirin and therefore, the risk of the medication surpasses its benefit in otherwise healthy women. Recent studies have shown that aspirin is important in preventing heart failure in patients with heart disease. All patients with heart disease should be on aspirin unless there are contraindications, such as bleeding problems.

Statins

Statins are the class of drugs used for lowering cholesterol. The common brand names on the market include: lovastatin (Mevacor), pravastatin (Pravachol), simvastatin (Zocor), fluvastatin (Lescol) atorvastatin (Lipitor), and rosuvastatin (Crestor). These drugs are used in preventing heart disease which can eventually lead to heart failure and have also been shown in recent studies to increase the survival in patients with diastolic heart failure where the heart has become stiff over a long period of time.

Dobutamine infusion

Patients who don't respond to standard therapy can sometimes benefit from the intravenous infusion of Dobutamine, a potent stimulant to heart contractility. It can only be given as a continuous IV drip and, therefore, is generally given over several days in the hospital. Sometimes it can be given at home with close in-home nursing supervision. Usually it is given in the hospital setting when the patient is admitted with an exacerbation of CHF. It can have deleterious effects on the heart in the long term and therefore its use should be limited.

Natrecor

Natrecor (nesiritide) was approved in 2001 for acute heart failure. It is a powerful intravenous treatment for hospitalized patients who are in florid heart failure and are not responding well to diuretics. Such patients have shortness of breath at rest or with minimal activity. Its use in outpatient settings is being assessed by the FDA for the treatment of chronic heart failure.

In summary, cardiologists use a combination of medication for the optimal treatment of heart failure. Not all medications will be used at their highest doses. Heart failure patients may notice that their regimen of drugs is not absolute and may differ from that of other patients.

4. Surgical and Non surgical Devices for CHF

External counterpulsation (ECP)

This well established non invasive treatment for angina is described in detail in Chapter 4. Recent research at the Orange County Heart Institute and several other centers has demonstrated a significant improvement in heart failure patients. Not only did symptoms improve but the weakened heart muscle showed a significant improvement in strength (the ejection fraction improved significantly). The treatment is the same as that for angina patients, that is 35 one-hour sessions, five days per week for seven weeks. Based on this research, our data was submitted to the FDA which gave approval for the treatment for congestive heart failure. However, as of this writing, Medicare has not approved reimbursement.

Inflatable cuffs are applied to the legs and inflate in a sequential manner to pump blood back to the heart during its the rest cycle. The cuffs sequentially deflate during the contraction phase of the heart, essentially making it easier for the heart to pump.

Biventricular Pacing

Using implanted cardiac pacemakers to treat congestive heart failure has been proposed as an adjunctive therapy. Initial results with standard two lead pacemaker systems have only been helpful in patients with dangerously low heart rates.

Recent observations and clinical studies have shown that electrical asynchrony has a significantly bad effect on cardiac performance and that this contributes to the poor pump performance in most patients with congestive heart failure. Electrical asynchrony can be diagnosed from the routine ECG obtained in your doctor's office. When asynchrony is present, a new pacing technique may be prescribed to resynchronize the heart and correct this problem. For many patients with congestive heart failure, re-synchronizing the heart can produce miraculous improvements.

Biventricular pacing or cardiac resynchronization therapy is the new pacing technique which corrects the electrical asynchrony and thereby strengthens the heart and improves symptoms in many patients with congestive heart failure. The technique of biventricular pacing is usually combined in a single device with an implantable defibrillator. This very sophisticated approach is called CRT-D or cardiac resynchronization therapy with defibrillation.

Like a standard pacemaker, the CRT system consists of a pulse generator connected to leads which go into the heart. The pulse generator is about the size of a deck of cards and is implanted under the skin in the upper chest. Wires or leads are then threaded into the heart via the major veins. CRT systems employ three leads instead of two in a standard pacemaker or defibrillator system. The third lead is placed via a large vein inside the heart, called the coronary sinus, and down one of the coronary sinus branches to pace the left ventricle. A standard lead is placed in the right ventricle and then both leads pace simultaneously to achieve biventricular pacing. The CRT system monitors the timing of the heart's contractions and can correct any abnormalities.

For many heart failure patients, cardiac resynchronization therapy improves quality of life and can prolong life. We have several patients who could barely walk across the room before CRT therapy and now are returning to a near normal lifestyle.

Most patients go home from the hospital within a day or two after the implant surgery and can return to regular activities within a few days.

This technique has been studied in many international multicenter randomized clinical trials which have shown significant benefits. Orange County Heart Institute has participated in several of the largest trials including the COMPANION and VECTOR clinical trials. During the course of these trials Orange County Heart Institute physicians implanted the first biventricular pacing systems in Orange County. To date, our physicians have implanted over 500 biventricular pacing systems.

The first patient implanted was GS, a 56-year-old white male with congestive heart failure and multiple prior heart attacks. Before implantation the patient could barely walk across the room without severe shortness of breath. After the new device was implanted he was able to return to a near normal activity level and his quality of life improved dramatically. A few weeks after the surgery, GS and his wife came into the office, gave us a hug and he told us "thanks for giving my life back to me."

Biventricular pacing is available now in most cardiology practices. Candidates for this therapy can be identified by changes on their ECG. Patients should ask their doctors if they are candidates for biventricular pacing.

Artificial Hearts and Assist Devices

Ever since Barney Clark received an artificial heart in the early 1980s in Salt Lake City, there have been hopes and expectations that modern medicine could develop such a device to replace a failing heart. Although a permanent, artificial replacement for the heart has not yet been successfully developed, there are devices which can temporarily support a failing heart. These devices are most commonly referred to as left ventricular assist devices (LVADs). In addition, there exist similar devices that will support both the right and left ventricles. They are called BiVADs (biventricular assist devices).

Left Ventricular Assist Devices

We occasionally use LVADs and BiVADs to support a failing heart after open-heart surgery. They are a form of "artificial heart" that actually pumps blood. These devices require surgical placement and intense cardiac monitoring in the intensive care unit. We leave them in place for several days while the failing heart regains strength. Hopefully, after just a few days the device can be removed and the heart will maintain blood pressure and cardiac output on its own. These devices should in no way be confused with an artificial heart that might sustain life for a long period of time in a natural setting. While attached to these devices, the patient is entirely bedridden and immobile, essentially on full life support. LVADs and BiVADs can also be used as a "bridge" to heart transplantation.

Heart Transplantation

Heart transplantation is an effective long term treatment for congestive heart failure. Most patients have a good long term outlook and often return to full and productive lives. However, due to the limited number of donor hearts, transplantation is a last resort and is reserved for the sickest of CHF patients. Those who have a very poor short term outlook where all of the above mentioned treatments have become ineffective and death is imminent receive the highest priority for transplant treatment.

In summary, congestive heart failure is a complex and sometimes difficult problem that affects millions of Americans. Although it used to be considered a terminal illness, CHF is currently manageable and most patients will improve substantially with appropriate therapy. Patients with this condition should seek out specialists in the area of heart failure management where advanced therapies can be employed to improve their lives. As a final effort, heart transplantation is used to treat end-stage CHF. Heart transplantation is obviously effective and proven. However, its use is limited by cost and the lack of adequate donors. It is also generally restricted to patients under 70 years of age and in otherwise good health.

7

Mitral Valve Prolapse and Heart Murmurs

M ary felt sharp stabbing chest pain off and on for several days before she saw the doctor. The pain would last only a few seconds at a time but was nonetheless worrisome to her. She also started to feel some skipping sensation, as if her heart stopped for a second. Her physician heard a heart murmur with his stethoscope and arranged for her to have an echocardiogram to further evaluate the murmur and to determine the cause of her symptoms. She was told that she had mitral valve prolapse (MVP). The doctor explained that the MVP was causing her chest pain and skipped beats and placed her on propranolol, a commonly used beta blocker class of medications which counter the effects of adrenaline on the heart. He also told her to take antibiotics to prevent the valve from getting infected during dental procedures. The doctor felt he diagnosed the cause of her symptoms; the patient was relieved that the symptoms were not in her head and she was given medications to control her MVP. That was in 1984. Echocardiograms were just becoming a common tool in medical practice at that time, and women were being diagnoised with a disease previously unheard of.

Mitral valve prolapse is the heart epidemic that never was. Referrals to cardiologists were soaring as more and more echocardiograms were being ordered to explain symptoms that in restropect were never due to the MVP or the MVP was mistakenly diagnosed. This did not occur because of bad medical practice. Instead, it was the state of the art approach with state of the art technology for a disease we did not fully understand. More and more women, especially in their 20s were given medicines for life, however most eventually stopped the meds on their own as their symptoms abated, but they were nevertheless labeled as "heart patients."

MVP is an over diagnosed condition. One estimate is that 10% of the women in the USA have MVP. In the vast majority of cases this is a benign condition.

The heart has four valves which act as one way doors so the blood travels in one direction as it flows through the four chambers of the heart. The two chambers on the top are called the atria and the two large pumping chambers on the bottom are the ventricles. Blood that returns from the body through the veins drains into the right atrium, then across the tricuspid valve into the right ventricle. The blood then flows across the pulmonic valve into the lungs where it receives oxygen. This oxygen rich blood drains into the left atrium, which then pumps the blood across the mitral valve, then into the main pumping chamber, the left ventricle, then the left ventricle pumps it across the aortic valve into the major artery of the body, the aorta, from which it travels to the head, muscle and all organs of the body.

The mitral valve is large and looks somewhat like a parachute. It is tethered in place by small fibrous cords. When the left ventricle contracts, the valve seals shut so the blood goes forward into the aorta, and not backward across the mitral valve into the left atrium.

MVP occurs when the mitral valve is a little larger than it should be and billows backward into the left atrium, or if the cords that are supposed to tether it in place are longer than they should be and the valve buckles or "prolapses" into the left atrium. When this happens, two things can occur:

1. The extra tissue of the valve prevents the valve from seating properly and the valve leaks. Small to moderate leakages of the valve are easily handled by the heart without obvious conse-

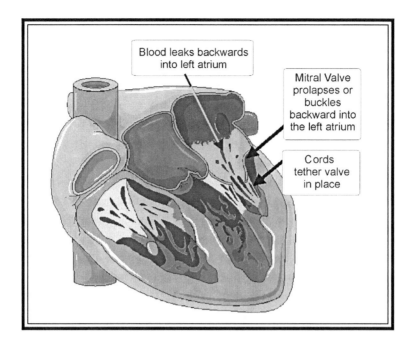

quences. But if there is moderate or more leakage, then the left ventricle will start to enlarge, eventually weaken and cause congestive heart failure, which can lead to significant shortness of breath;

2. When the valve prolapses a lot, extra tension is placed on the cords which on one end are attached to the inner surface of the heart muscle of the left ventricle. Sometimes enough strain is placed on the cords that they can eventually snap and cause the valve to flail backwards, causing significant leakage. If the valve leaks a tremendous amount, then blood does not drain out of the lungs and sudden shortness of breath and eventual congestive heart failure occurs and the valve needs to be surgically repaired. The valve may be slightly more prone to infection, a condition called endocarditis. Most of these infections, though extremely rare, occur from dental work. However, even if there is significant prolapse of the valve and leakage of blood, antibiotics are no longer recommended before dental work.

The bottom line on MVP: Those who are now properly diagnosed have a 99% chance of having no significant problems.

With strict diagnostic criteria and newer echocardiographic machines, MVP is much less common than the 10% previously reported. Here are some findings:

• Those who are now properly diagnosed have a 99% chance of having no significant problems.

• The key is how much the valve leaks. If it is severe it can cause problems that may require the valve to be surgically repaired.

• It is very unlikely that chest pain and palpitations are due to the prolapsing valve and usually medications are not needed.

• If the valve prolapses and leaks at least a moderate amount, then the valve may be more prone to infection during dental procedures. However, antibiotics are no longer deemed beneficial and are not recommended before any dental work.

• If you were diagnosed with MVP more than five years ago, you should see a cardiologist and be reevaluated with a newer echocardiogram machine to see if you do or do not have MVP and if any medications should be stopped.

Heart Murmurs

A heart murmur is simply a sound coming from the heart as blood flows through the chambers. A stethoscope is needed to hear most heart murmurs. Most are benign, also referred to as "innocent murmurs." They are not dangerous in any way. An innocent murmur means that the murmur is not due to a significant leakage or narrowing of the heart valves nor is it due to holes between the chambers of the heart. It is simply due to the normal flow of blood through the heart chambers. Heart murmurs can also get louder or softer depending on the heart rate or the amount of fluid in the body (some murmurs may get louder or softer if you are dehydrated). Pathological murmurs are those that are due to deformed valves that leak or are narrowed (or both), or to a hole between the chambers of the heart.

The best way to diagnose a murmur is with an exam by a cardiologist and an evaluation with echocardiogram. The two most important valves are the aortic and the mitral, both on the left side of the heart. A narrowing of the valve is called stenosis. Leaking of a heart valve is called regurgitation or insufficiency. Congenital holes between the chambers of the heart also cause murmurs and make the heart prone to infection. These congenital abnormalities are referred to as atrial septal defects (a hole between the top chambers, the atria), or ventricular septal defects (a hole between the bottom chambers, the ventricles). The vast majority of deformed or defective valves have only a mild degree of narrowing or restriction and thus can be followed and treated medically. These valves very likely never need surgical repair. Severe conditions can successfully be treated with replacement by artificial valves. Antibiotics are no longer recommended prior to dental work for any heart murmur or abnormal heart valve. However, if a person has had heart surgery and has had an artificial heart valve replacement, then antibiotics are still required.

The bottom line on heart murmurs: Ninety percent of all murmurs are harmless and will never lead to a clinical problem. Echocardiograms are needed to fully evaluate the significance of the murmur if on physical exam the murmur suggests the valve is deformed.

8

Heart Valve Disease

Valves of the Heart

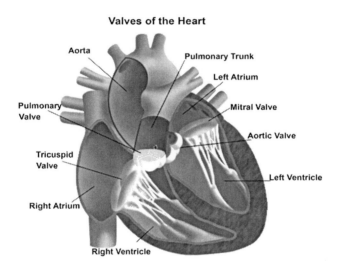

The human heart is two pumps connected in series by tubing but physically housed together with a common power source, creating a very efficient design. Each pump unit is composed of a smaller atrium on top and a larger ventricle on the bottom. The atria and ventricles are separated by valves, the mitral valve on the left and the tricuspid valve on the right. The ventricles then pump blood into arteries and are separated from the arteries by valves, the aortic valve on the left and the pulmonic valve on the right. The four valves act as one way doors so the blood travels in one direction as it flows through the four chambers of the heart. Blood that returns from the body through the veins drains to the right atrium, then across the tricuspid valve into the right ventricle then across the pulmonic valve into the lungs where it receives oxygen. This oxygen rich blood drains into the left atrium which then pumps the blood across the mitral valve into the main pumping chamber, the left ventricle; then the left ventricle pumps it across the aortic valve into the major artery of the body, the aorta, where it travels to the head, muscle and all organs of the body.

Types of valve disease: Does the valve leak or is it narrowed?

A valve can become narrowed, which is referred to as "stenosis," or it can leak blood backwards through the heart chambers; this is referred to as "regurgitation" or "insufficiency." When symptoms of chest pain, shortness of breath or loss of consciousness occur, and the appropriate physical exam findings, echocardiographic findings and cardiac catheterization findings are all consistent with a severe stenosis, then repair or replacement of the valve is needed.

When a valve leaks a great deal, symptoms may not be a reliable indicator because the heart may be significantly enlarged or weakened from the extra burden of the leaky valve *before* symptoms occur. Then, surgical treatment may not be beneficial because the heart is too weakened. So with a leaky valve, physical examination and echocardiograms are required to determine when the heart *starts* to enlarge or weaken, so that the valve can be repaired or replaced even if there are no symptoms. The results are usually very good, with excellent long term outcomes when the valve surgery is properly timed.

Is one valve more important than another?

In general, the two valves on the left side of the heart, the mitral and aortic valve, are far more important than the two valves on the right side of the heart, the tricuspid and pulmonic valves.

The reason is that the mitral and aortic valves are under much higher pressure than the right sided valves. The left sided valves are responsible for getting the blood out to the whole body, and are therefore subject to the pressure in our arteries, that is, our blood pressure, which is normally, for systolic pressure, around 100 to 140 mm Hg. Whereas, the right sided valves pump blood into the lungs. The pressure in the lungs is usually only about 30mm Hg, much lower of course than our blood pressure.

So, in general, the aortic valve and mitral valve are much more likely to fail, and when they do fail, the consequences are greater compared to the tricsupid and pulmonic valves. In addition, aortic and mitral valve disease is many times more common than right sided valve disease.

The Mitral Valve

The mitral valve is a large bicuspid valve that looks somewhat like a parachute. It is tethered in place by small fibrous cords secured to muscular bundles in the left ventricle called papillary muscles. When the ventricle contracts, the valve seals shut so the blood goes forward into the aorta, and not backward across the mitral valve into the left atrium. When the ventricle relaxes during the diastolic phase of the cardiac cycle, the valve opens and blood goes from the left atrium into the left ventricle.

Mitral Valve Regurgitation

Mitral regurgitation (MR) occurs when the mitral valve leaks or becomes incompetent. When the left ventricle contracts, instead of closing and blocking flow from the ventricle into the atrium, the valve leaks and blood flows backward into the atrium. The larger the leak, the more serious the consequences. Mitral regurgitation produces dilation of the left atrium due to volume overload. MR can occur due to aging, or to blocked coronary arteries which cause a heart attack and damage the attachment of the valve to the heart. Also, any condition that causes the left ventricle to enlarge or weaken can cause the valve to be stretched out and not close properly. In such cases, improving the function of the ventricle and causing it to shrink toward normal size, often will reduce the leakage of the mitral valve. Other conditions, like connective tissue disease, arthritic conditions, infection and trauma can also cause the valve to leak, but are far less common.

Mild MR generally requires no treatment, but as the MR increases, treatment may be helpful. Typical symptoms include shortness of breath, fatigue, palpitations, chest pain and even congestive heart failure. Fluid may accumulate in the legs and abdomen. Patients with MR also have a very distinctive murmur and should have echocardiograms to quantitate the degree of insufficiency. Medical management with diuretics and/or drugs that reduce blood pressure are the mainstay of medical management. Typical medications are ACE inhibitors (angiotensin converting enzyme inhibitors) and ARBs (ACE receptor blockers). In cases of severe mitral regurgitation, open heart surgery may be necessary to repair or replace the valve.

Mitral Valve Stenosis

Mitral stenosis refers to abnormal thickening and consequent narrowing of the valve orifice in the mitral position between the left atrium and left ventricle. The most common cause of mitral stenosis is rheumatic fever. However mitral stenosis can be congenital, occur as a complication of carcinoid syndrome or be associated with systemic lupus erythematosus and rheumatoid arthritis.

The normal mitral valve orifice is four to six square centimeters. When the valve area falls to roughly half that figure it is considered stenotic. The consequences of mitral stenosis are enlargement of the left atrium due to elevation of pressure above the stenotic valve. The more severe the obstruction, the more severe the problems. Arrhythmias such as atrial fibrillation are very common and congestive heart failure may occur. The most common symptom is shortness of breath. Chest pain, coughing especially with blood, hoarseness due to the enlarged atrium compressing the voice box, enlargement of the liver and abdomen and swelling of the legs are all common features of mitral stenosis.

Mitral stenosis can be easily diagnosed by a thorough physical exam. Mitral stenosis produces a classic heart murmur which any good cardiologist should hear. In any patient suspected of mitral stenosis, an echocardiogram should be performed to verify the diagnosis and directly visualize the valve. All patients with mitral stenosis or any other valve abnormality should receive antibiotics prior to dental work to protect against heart valve infection. Diuretics are usually required to reduce congestion and ultimately many patients will require open heart surgery to repair or replace the stenotic valve.

The Aortic Valve

The aortic valve separates the left ventricle from the aorta and is the valve which regulates flow to the entire body. When the valve becomes narrowed or blocked it is stenotic. Aortic stenosis is a relatively common valve disorder and therefore presents a major clinical challenge.

Aortic Valve Stenosis

Normally the aortic valve has three leaflets, however congenital malformations in which the valve is bileaflet or has a small malformed third leaflet are common. Deformed congenital bileaflet aortic valve is the most common cause of aortic stenosis in this country. When we are young, the valve, even though deformed with only two leaflets, is still quite flexible and causes no restriction to blood flow. Then over the years, the wear and tear of blood flowing across the deformed valve cause calcium build up and scar tissue to develop, restricting the opening of the valve. These patients may be fine for most of their lives and then present at age 50 or 60 with stenosis of the valve. Aortic stenosis may also occur due to rheumatic heart disease and is sometimes seen in conjunction with mitral stenosis.

Aortic stenosis is also associated with a typical heart murmur and can be verified by echocardiography. Physiologically, aortic stenosis produces a dilation of the left ventricle and impaired forward flow of blood. This can cause chest pain, fainting spells and ultimately congestive heart failure. In cases of mild stenosis medical therapy with diuretics may be all that is necessary. In cases of severe aortic stenosis the best treatment is to relieve the blockage. This can be achieved temporarily by dilating the valve with a balloon. Permanent relief can only be obtained by open heart surgery and replacement of the valve.

Aortic Valve Regurgitation

Insufficiency of the aortic valve results in backward regurgitation of blood into the left ventricle after contraction and ejection of blood out of the left ventricle into the aorta. This may result from intrinsic structural abnormalities of the valve apparatus or the ascending aorta or both. Rheumatic aortic valve disease, congenital abnormalities of the valve, trauma, infection, collagen vascular diseases especially Marfans syndrome, syphilis and aging can all produce insufficiency of the aortic valve. Similar to mitral regurgitation, this results in a volume overload condition.

More commonly however, AR is a chronic process and the patient experiences an uncomfortable awareness of the heart beating forcefully in the chest and neck. Inspection of the patient may reveal a nodding of the head with every heartbeat which is called De Mussetts sign and was originally described hundreds of years ago in syphilitic patients. In any case, AR is associated with a typical diastolic murmur (a murmur that occurs during the rest cycle of the heart beat) and can be confirmed and quantified by echocardiography. Mild cases can be treated with observation or medically with diuretics and blood pressure control. More severe cases may require repair or replacement of the aortic valve.

Tricuspid, pulmonic and multivavular disease

Tricuspid regurgitation (TR) is very common, and mild degrees are often seen with perfectly normal hearts and may never cause a problem. It is also commonly seen in conditions associated with dilation of the right ventricle. This is seen in right ventricular failure of any kind, usually due to chronic lung disease which makes it more difficult for the right ventricle to pump blood into the lungs.

TR is generally well tolerated but when associated with lung problems and pulmonary hypertension (increased pressure in the artery leading to the lung) it can lead to shortness of breath, fatigue and congestive heart failure. Other conditions that can cause tricuspid regurgitation are carcinoid syndrome, pulmonary hypertension and thyroid disease. TR has a typical murmur and should be evaluated with echocardiography.

Tricuspid valve stenosis (TS) is rare, is almost always associated with rheumatic fever and is generally accompanied by mitral stenosis. The fundamental approach to TS is surgical replacement of the valve. In patients with congestive heart failure, diuretics and salt and fluid restriction are required.

Pulmonary valve problems are usually congenital. Pulmonary regurgitation, although rare, may occur with dilation of the right ventricle and is most commonly seen as a manifestation of carcinoid. Pulmonary stenosis is always a congenital problem and generally presents in infancy.

Cardiac Valve Surgery

Any malfunctioning valve may need to be repaired or replaced. The degree of narrowing (stenosis) or insufficiency (regurgitation) and the patient's clinical status will determine the need for valve surgery.

A narrowed mitral valve may be opened with a balloon in a nonsurgical catheter procedure done by a cardiologist in an X-ray suite or catheterization laboratory. The patient needs light sedation while the doctor threads the balloon catheter through the artery of the leg into the heart and then across the narrowed valve. The balloon is then inflated to open the narrowing. Unfortunately this procedure provides only temporary relief. The balloon procedure lasts longer for mitral stenosis than it does for aortic valve stenosis.

The procedure, called balloon valvuloplasty, is best reserved for patients with mild to moderate narrowing or those who are too frail to undergo open heart surgery.

Repair of a damaged valve is always preferable to actual replacement, but it may not be possible if the valve is severely damaged and deformed. Repair of the valve is truly an art performed by an experienced surgeon during open heart surgery. The surgeon will attempt to reconstruct the valve from native valve tissue while the patient is under general anesthesia and on the heart-lung bypass machine.

Replacement of the valve is frequently necessary. Prosthetic valves are composed of metal and/or plastic and other synthetic materials. The valves are durable and will usually last for the life of the patient. The main disadvantage of prosthetic valves is that they are associated with the development of blood clots on the synthetic material. Blood thinners such as warfarin or coumadin will be prescribed to prevent this problem. Tissue valves are composed of natural materials from cows, pigs or human materials. Tissue valves are not as durable as prosthetic valves, usually lasting less than ten years. The main advantage of the tissue valve is that it does not cause blood clots, and therefore will not require blood thinning drug therapy.

Each approach to valve problems has particular risks and benefits so it is important to discuss the alternatives thoroughly with your cardiologist and cardiac surgeon. At the Orange County Heart Institute, it is our practice to routinely discuss all valve cases in a combined cardiology-cardiac surgery conference in which the entire team is present. All the options are considered and we then present the results of our conference and our final recommendations to the patient.

9

Palpitations
and
Abnormal Heart Rhythms

Abnormalities of the heart's electrical rhythm are called arrhythmias. Pay strict attention if your heartbeat feels unusual. Arrhythmias are frequently seen in women of all ages. The most feared risk of arrhythmia is sudden death, or sudden electrical failure of the heart. At this writing, sudden death will kill more Americans than all cancers combined, and the risk is greater for women. Why are women at increased risk? The answer is unknown but may be related to the complex hormonal physiology of women. Studies have shown that female hormones may produce arrhythmia by affecting potassium and calcium ion channels which regulate the heart's electrical rhythm. So, exactly what are arrhythmias in a woman's heart?

Overview

Your heart works like a pump you might buy in a hardware store because it is powered by electricity. Everybody is born with an electric generator or pacemaker in the heart called the sinoatrial node. The heart is wired to transmit the electric impulse over the entire surface. The wiring is called the atrioventricular node and His-Purkinje system.

A single electric impulse initiates each heartbeat. At rest, a normal woman will have 60 to 80 heartbeats per minute. If the heart rate goes too slow (bradyarrhythmias) or too fast (tachyarrhythmias), then serious problems can develop and prompt therapy is required. Arrhythmias lead to a number of serious symptoms including palpitation, dizzy spells, fainting, fatigue, and sudden death. Palpitation is the most frequent symptom and refers to the sensation of skipped beats, extra beats or the sensation of a rapid heartbeat.

Unfortunately, in women these symptoms are often ascribed to monthly hormonal changes, stress or emotional problems, when in fact there is an underlying heart condition.

B.T. was a 32-year-old black woman referred for evaluation of palpations. She had previously been diagnosed with an anxiety disorder and placed on Valium, but the drug did not alleviate her symptoms and caused lethargy and fatigue. She was disabled by her condition and the side effects of the Valium and had to quit working. Subsequently she underwent evaluation at the Orange County Heart Institute and was diagnosed with arrhythmia and treated with ablation therapy which cured her problem. She was able to return to her career in teaching and is doing well today.

Types of Arrhythmia

1. Atrial Fibrillation

Atrial fibrillation (AF) is the most common cardiac arrhythmia. This year, one million new cases of atrial fibrillation will occur in the United States and most will be in women. AF is characterized by a lack of contraction of the atrium which fibrillates (quivers) without effectively contracting and propelling blood forward.

Although atrial fibrillation can occur in otherwise healthy people, it is often associated with some other cardiovascular condition: hypertension, congestive heart failure, mitral valve disease, and coronary artery disease. It commonly occurs following bypass surgery and can also be caused by a number of non-cardiac conditions such as infection, inflammatory disease, thyroid problems and emotional stress.

Complications of atrial fibrillation

1. Symptoms related to low output of the heart: fatigue, breathlessness and congestive heart failure. Because the atrium just quivers and fails to contract in a unified manner, the heart does not pump blood as efficiently as it should. There may be a 20 to 40% fall in heart pump effectiveness. This can cause fatigue or decreased exercise capacity, and may aggravate congestive heart failure. Sometimes the electrical activity of the fibrillating atrium can drive the ventricle to beat far too fast and quite irregularly. This can cause low blood pressure, reduced functional capacity, fatigue, shortness of breath and depression.

2. Clots forming in the left atrium that may lead to a stroke. Because the atrium is not contracting, the blood may pool in the atrium and form clots. If a clot travels to the brain, it can cause a stroke. The incidence of stroke in women patients with atrial fibrillation is about two to four percent per year.

Treatment of atrial fibrillation: rhythm control and stroke prevention

1. Rhythm control

The immediate treatment goal in AF is to regulate the ventricular response rate so the heart slows to less than one hundred beats per minute. We achieve this by administering medications such as digoxin, cardizem, verapamil or beta blockers.

The next goal is to convert the heart back to a regular rhythm. We achieve this with anti-arrhythmic medications or with electrical cardioversion.

If treated within one to two days of onset, we can perform a cardioversion without risk of a stroke. If the patient has been in atrial fibrillation for more than a few days, then he or she must be treated with coumadin for two to four weeks to dissolve any possible clot prior to cardioversion.

The presence or absence of a clot in the atrium can be assessed by doing a transesophageal echocardiogram (TEE). See Chapter 1 for a full discussion of TEE. A TEE can also help predict the risk of stroke.

Catheter Ablation

More recently, new technology has been developed to allow atrial fibrillation to be cured with catheter ablation, an outpatient procedure with light sedation and local anesthetic and without surgery. It involves placing catheters into the heart through the veins of the legs. Selected areas in the heart are then cauterized, or ablated, using high frequency radio waves to generate the heat. The ablation is actually painless because there are no nerve endings in the heart. Currently, the Orange County Heart Institute performs 300 to 400 ablation procedures annually without major complications. Cure rates for AF are 70 to 80% and 98% for other atrial arrhythmias. After the ablation, which takes from one to four hours, patients need to stay flat in bed for approximately four hours and then are up and around. Ablation patients are usually monitored in the hospital overnight and then sent home the next morning. The patients should then have a light day and on the following day can return to their usual activities.

The MAZE procedure is another type of ablation that is done only at the time of open heart surgery when a patient is undergoing coronary bypass or replacement of a heart valve. The surgeon makes partial cuts through the inner surface of the atrium to stop the abnormal electrical activity that is causing the atrial fibrillation. The MAZE procedure is never done as a stand-alone procedure by itself to cure atrial fibrillation since it requires opening the heart chambers and the alternative catheter-based ablation is so much less invasive.

Cardioversion

When your heartbeat is irregular, medicine is often used first. If that does not work, cardioversion may be the next step. Here is what happens. Your cardiologist administers a small, brief, electric shock while you are asleep. The shock helps your heartbeat return to normal. A cardioversion is performed in a hospital, and you will be there from two to four hours.

Beforehand, be sure to tell the doctor what medicines you take. He or she may ask you to take blood thinners for a few weeks prior to the cardioversion.

Risks are minimal. Orange County Heart Institute physicians have performed over 1,500 cardioversion procedures without complications.

2. Preventing a stroke

Coumadin is the most effective drug to prevent a stroke from atrial fibrillation, though there are certain patients who do just as well with aspirin, as discussed earlier.

A new method of stroke prevention for patients with atrial fibrillation uses heart catheterization techniques to deliver a filter (WATCHMAN device) into the appendage of the left atrium where clots appear to develop (See figure). Once installed, the filter prevents stroke by blocking migration of the clots out of the appendage. This procedure is available at the Orange County Heart Institute on an investigational basis. Mary B. is a 68-year-

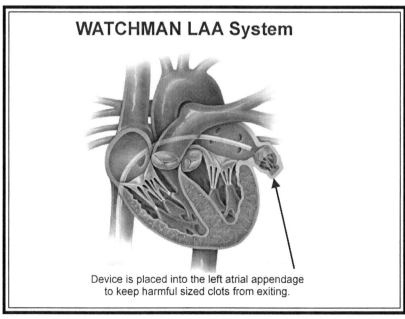

WATCHMAN LAA System

Device is placed into the left atrial appendage
to keep harmful sized clots from exiting.

old woman with atrial fibrillation who was prescribed Coumadin to prevent stroke. She subsequently was referred and underwent the WATCHMAN device implant and has been able to permanently stop her Coumadin.

Chronic atrial fibrillation

Many patients cannot achieve or maintain a regular heart rhythm and may be chronically in atrial fibrillation for the rest of their lives. This occurs in approximately half of all patients with atrial fibrillation. In these cases, we give medications such as digoxin and cardizem to control the heart rate. Coumadin or aspirin is prescribed to reduce the risk of stroke. The WATCHMAN device is also indicated for chronic atrial fibrillation.

Sometimes the medications cannot effectively control the rapid heart rate without causing the heart to "pause" or go too slow. This syndrome has been called a tachy-brady syndrome due to the alternating rapid and slow heart rates. In these cases, we place a pacemaker to prevent slow heart rates, and a catheter ablation of the electrical connection between the atrium and ventricle (AV node) to prevent rapid heart rates. This prevents the quivering atrium from driving the ventricle too rapidly and irregularly.

2. Premature contractions

Common causes of palpitations are PVCs (premature ventricular contractions) and PACs (premature atrial contractions). These are single extra beats. PVCs produce a pause in the heartbeat, often followed by a thump or unusually strong beat. PACs produce a sensation of an extra beat. PVCs and PACs are commonly felt at nighttime when one is relaxed and rested.

PVCs and PACs often occur in healthy people with no evident heart disease. They can occur in response to an excess of caffeine or other stimulants and can also occur in patients who have left-ventricular hypertrophy (thickened heart muscle) in response to high blood pressure.

Though often disconcerting to patients, PACs and PVCs are of very little medical importance and rarely pose any risk. Premature beats are not dangerous, just bothersome. In rare cases, PVCs and PACs can indicate more serious heart problems such as hypertension or coronary artery disease and they can cause fatigue and lightheadedness if they occur as frequently as every second or third beat.

Cause of PVCs and PACs

Premature contractions are caused by an abnormal electrical activity within the atrium or ventricle that causes the heart to beat and contract earlier than normal. It contracts so early that it has not had time to fill with blood during diastole, the relaxation or filling phase of the cardiac cycle. When the heart contracts half empty, it creates an absent or weak pulse in the heart rate perceived by the patient.

Premature contractions can occur commonly in people who have long-standing high blood pressure, valvular heart disease, or coronary artery disease. They also can occur as a result of stimulants such as caffeine, alcohol, or medications taken by asthma patients. Stress also probably has a role in the development of arrhythmias. Unfortunately stress is difficult to quantify. There is no unit of measure for stress like inches or yards. But certainly we would recommend reduction of stress to patients with symptomatic PVCs. Methods such as biofeedback, meditation, and exercise may be helpful, but there is no magic pill to reduce stress.

Since premature contractions rarely present any risk, it is best not to treat them with antiarrhythmic medications. Treatment can be expensive and dangerous. Common medications such as Procan SR, Quinaglute, Rhythmol, Betapace, and others are costly and more important, they can cause life-threatening side effects.

Patients with extreme symptoms may require suppression of the arrhythmia. In these cases, the safest and most effective treatment is to undergo an electrophysiologic study. The cardiologist can identify the source of the premature contraction using new state of the art intracardiac mapping techniques in which catheters are placed into the heart. If there is a single source, then an ablation can be performed. The area ablated is usually only a few millimeters in diameter.

Gail B. is a 34-year-old white woman who presented with debilitating palpitations which she described as skipped beats and then hard beats often associated with a choking sensation. An outpatient ECG documented PVCs as the cause of her symptoms. She subsequently underwent successful radiofrequency ablation at the Orange County Heart Institute and is now symptom free.

3. Supraventricular tachycardia (SVT)

SVT refers to any arrhythmia coming from above the ventricle. SVT includes reentrant paroxysmal supraventricular tachycardia (PSVT), true atrial tachycardias, atrial fibrillation and atrial flutter. True atrial tachycardias are arrhythmias that arise from an abnormal site in the atrium that leads to uncontrolled, rapid electrical stimulation of the heart. This may be called ectopic atrial tachycardia or paroxysmal atrial tachycardia (PAT). PAT accounts for approximately five percent of all SVT. Reentrant SVT is much more common and is caused by a second abnormal electrical connection between the atrium and ventricle which then short circuits the heart, causing paroxysmal rapid heart rate. This second abnormal electrical pathway may be a second atrioventricular nodal (AV) pathway or may be outside the AV node. This complex rhythm is caused by electrical activity that travels down from the atrium to the ventricle usually via the normal electrical pathway, and then inappropriately goes backward into the atrium via the second accessory abnormal pathway. We refer to this as a "circus movement." This rhythm happens when the electricity creates a pathway resembling a circle under a circus tent.

Symptoms of SVT
SVT causes a rapid heartbeat. Often this is described as a feeling of the heart beating rapidly, pounding, or the sensation of

palpitations. It can be associated with chest pain, anxiety, dizziness or fainting. Most cases of SVT are caused by a congenital second abnormal electrical pathway in the heart. Symptoms usually begin in the teens but can occur at any age.

We have seen one patient who had no problems until she was 84 years old. At that time, her heart started racing and she was initially diagnosed with panic disorder. Subsequently a more thorough evaluation was undertaken and SVT was discovered. She underwent successful ablation therapy at the Orange County Heart Institute and was cured of her problem. For years, many doctors have inappropriately told patients that they were experiencing "panic attacks" when in fact their problem is a more serious heart condition. Often SVT is attributed to mitral valve prolapse when in fact there is no relationship between the two. We have seen many other young women with recurrent SVT who have been misdiagnosed with panic attacks or other emotional problems when in fact they have a curable heart problem. Because SVT may be triggered by elevated hormone levels, symptoms often occur during the menstrual cycle or with pregnancy and this leads to misdiagnosis. In reality, they have been suffering from SVT that caused them to panic from the abnormal sensation. Treatment of the SVT eliminates the "panic attacks."

Treatment of SVT

We can treat SVT with medications such as digoxin, beta blockers, or anti-arrhythmic medications. However, since these conditions are usually recurrent and require medical therapy for life, and since the medications are not always effective, cause side effects, and can be expensive, it is often better to eliminate these rhythms permanently by performing an ablation.

Ablation of tachy-arrhythmias (fast heart rhythms)

Tachy-arrhythmias are episodes during which the heart rhythm is too fast. These can be triggered by a variety of factors. Often, they occur due to an electrical "short circuit" within the heart. This causes the heart to race spontaneously until the electrical pathway resumes its normal course. Sometimes tachycardia occurs with a normal heart rhythm. These fast normal rhythms (sinus tachycardia) are driven by anxiety, stimulants, fever, anemia, or other noncardiac causes.

When medications are considered inadequate or ineffective, the cardiologist will consider doing an electrophysiologic (EP) study to try to reproduce the tachy-arrhythmia in a controlled setting, then identify where it is coming from.

Performance of an EP study requires a visit to the catheterization lab. Light sedation is used to keep the patient comfortable. After the skin is numbed with local anesthesia, a puncture is made and a sheath placed in a large vein. Catheters are then advanced into the heart under fluoroscopy. Once positioned, these catheters can map the electrical conduction and attempt to stimulate or reproduce the abnormal rhythm. Once the source of the abnormal rhythm is identified, it can often be cured or eliminated through an ablation. The scar tissue from the procedure eliminates the source of the arrhythmia.

These procedures are usually performed on an outpatient basis.

Complications can include bleeding at the puncture site. Rarely, an EP study or ablation can cause "heart block" that requires placement of a pacemaker. This occurs less than one percent of the time. Other complications can include a puncture of the heart with a catheter. Again, this is rare and usually not serious, but it could require surgery to repair. An EP study and ablation carry a very low risk of complication.

Breaking a rapid heart rhythm

If otherwise healthy patients spontaneously develop rapid, regular heart rates, they may have gone into a SVT. Such fast heartbeats can be broken and returned to normal by stimulating the vagus nerve, which slows the heart. The vagus nerve is stimulated in three ways: massaging the carotid artery, sudden ice-water (facial) immersion, or the Valsalva maneuver, which is bearing down and pushing with the abdominal muscles.

4. Brady-arrhythmias (slow heart rates)

Brady-arrhythmias are heart rhythms that are too slow or have intermittent long pauses. Brady-arrhythmias may arise at the level of the sinus node or main pacemaker of the heart or lower down in the electrical connections between the atrium and the ventricle.

Sick sinus syndrome

Sick sinus syndrome (SSS) refers to problems originating in the sinus node or main pacemaker of the heart. When the sinus node does not function properly, slow heart rates result.

The most common cause of SSS is degeneration due to aging, but problems may also result from lack of adequate blood flow (ischemia), trauma or toxins such as excessive alcohol. Treatment of SSS can not be achieved with any medication and requires a replacement of the sinus node with a permanent pacemaker.

Heart Block

Heart block refers to block of electrical conduction from the atrium through the atrioventricular node to the ventricles. In this situation, the sinus node or pacemaker of the heart is firing impulses but these impulses are not reaching their destination due to damage or malfunction of the electrical connection. This electrical block results in failure of the heart to contract and slower heart rates.

Calcification of the heart's electrical conduction system

Calcification of the heart's electrical system can lead to problems including severe slow heart rates producing dizziness, fatigue, fainting or sudden death. Simple age or degeneration is the cause of this condition. Calcification of the heart tissues invades the electrical conduction tissues and blocks proper transmission of impulses from the atrium to the ventricle.

Ischemia

Coronary artery plaques or myocardial infarction can limit blood flow to the heart's conduction system, causing damage and consequently heart rates that are too slow. These conditions often cause heart block.

Brady-arrhythmias may improve simply by avoiding medications that aggravate the situation, including digitalis, beta blockers and certain calcium channel blockers. Elderly patients, especially women with smaller body mass, are very sensitive to these medicines. At the Orange County Heart Institute, we try to avoid combinations of these medicines and use half the usual dose for our elderly female patients.

Symptoms of Brady-Arrhythmias

Generally, a heart rate that is too slow to provide adequate blood flow to the brain will make a person lightheaded or dizzy. It can sometimes result in loss of consciousness and fainting. Bradycardia can rarely result in a sudden arrest of the heart or sudden death and therefore should be treated as an emergency. Unexplained bradycardia especially with a wide complex rhythm should be treated as hyperkalemia (elevated potassium level) until proven otherwise.

Treatment: Pacemakers

The usual treatment for symptomatic slow heart rhythms or pauses is to have a pacemaker implanted. Pacemakers have existed for over twenty years and have become increasingly smaller and more sophisticated. They represent a truly amazing blend of medical need and electrical engineering which monitor the heart and stimulate it to beat if its rate becomes too slow. Currently, they are about the size of two or three silver dollars in a stack.

Pacemakers are usually implanted under the skin just below the collarbone. They are attached to the heart via one or two leads attached to the atrium and ventricle of the heart via a vein. The pacemaker system is composed of a pulse generator and insulated wires or leads. These devices are reliable and have a battery life from five to ten years. Battery replacement requires re-

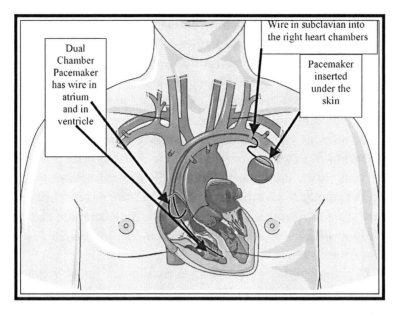

moval of the actual pacemaker pulse generator and replacement with a new unit. Pre-existing lead wires that connect the pulse generator to the heart tissue will usually last for the life of the patient.

An incision about two inches in length is made to implant the pacemaker. A pocket for it is carefully made between the skin and muscle. A needle then enters the subclavian vein under the clavicle. Into the vein are passed one or two pacemaker leads. These leads are passed into the right ventricle and right atrium. The leads attach permanently to the heart via a screw or via little flanges or tines that press against the heart tissue and become strongly fixed in place.

The pacemaker leads are attached to the generator and the pocket is then sutured and closed. The patient is observed on a cardiac monitor for twelve to twenty-four hours and then sent home.

Potential complications include infection, bleeding and collapsed lung. Although serious, these complications are quite rare, occurring in only one to two percent of all cases.

As pacemakers continue to get "smarter" and smaller each year, they are not cheap. They cost between $3,000 and $6,000. The cardiologist's fee for implantation is usually about $1,000.

Pacemakers have to be monitored to insure that they are properly adjusted to your heart condition. The electrical output and sensing mechanisms are adjusted to use the least amount of energy possible, thereby prolonging the battery life. You will usually see the cardiologist every three to six months to check the battery and adjust the pacemaker.

On average, pacemakers last five to ten years before the battery expires. Since the battery is built into the generator as a solid-state unit, when the battery expires, the entire unit must be replaced. Usually, the leads that go from the pacemaker to the heart tissue are still usable and do not require replacement. The new generator with the new battery is implanted and attached to the preexisting leads.

In patients who have had a pacemaker for many years, the leads may become old and cracked, or their insulation may become frayed. The leads are no longer useful, but since they are attached firmly to the inside of the heart, they are not easily removed. Often, one or two defective leads will be left in place while new leads are placed alongside them. However, with time, as more and more leads accumulate, the old leads need to be removed. They can be a potential source of infection or of a clot in the major veins leading to the heart.

The best extraction technique, recently developed, uses a Spectranetics excimer laser to remove the old leads. The laser device is passed down and around the old lead, freeing it from the scar tissue, allowing it to be safely removed. Not all hospitals have an excimer laser but this technique should be sought by interested patients. Laser lead extractions are routinely available through the Orange County Heart Institute.

5. *Ventricular Tachycardia/Fibrillation*

Ventricular tachycardia and fibrillation are related arrhythmias occurring generally in the setting of serious heart problems or cardiomyopathy. Ventricular tachycardia is a rhythm originating from abnormal electrical circuits within the ventricle. It is usually rapid (greater than 150 beats/minute) and therefore causes ineffective heart-muscle pumping. It can cause low blood pressure and blackout spells. It can also degenerate into life-threatening ventricular fibrillation.

Ventricular fibrillation is the ineffectual quivering of the ventricle. It causes no effective blood flow and leads to permanent brain damage and death within a few minutes. Virtually all patients with VF will have damaged heart muscle from an acute or previous heart attack or cardiomyopathy.

Fast Fact
Arrhythmia leading to sudden death kills more people than all cancers combined— nearly one person every minute! Women are at particularly high risk.

Sudden cardiac death (SCD) from a sustained ventricular tachycardia or fibrillation is in fact the most common form of death in the United States. Arrhythmia leading to sudden death kills more people than all cancers combined, nearly one person every minute! Women are at particularly high risk. In fact, more women than men will die suddenly this year. Patients at risk for SCD have a weak heart usually from a heart attack but also possibly from hypertension, viral infection or excessive alcohol intake. Most patients who have required coronary artery bypass surgery have had some damage to their heart and these patients may also be at risk for sudden cardiac death. The strength or weakness of the heart can be measured by an echocardiogram (ultrasound) of the heart which we routinely perform in our offices at the Orange County Heart Institute. The test takes about 15 minutes and the results are available immediately. The strength of the heart is reported as the *ejection fraction,* which is the percentage of blood in the heart pumped out with one contraction. A normal ejection fraction is 60 to 70%. When the ejection fraction falls below 40%, the risk of sudden death is high enough to warrant further studies and treatment. The only effective therapy to prevent sudden death is an automatic implantable cardioverter-defibrillator (AICD), the device Vice President Richard Cheney received prophylactically to prevent sudden death. He was without any specific symptoms of arrhythmia but his doctors felt he needed the device to prevent sudden death simply because his heart was weak. This approach has been scientifically shown to prolong and improve life in several large multi-center international randomized clinical trials including the MADIT, MUSST, and AVID trials. The Orange County Heart Institute was privileged to participate in many of these trials and currently AICDs are routinely implanted in hundreds of patients each year at our center.

Treatment: Automatic implantable defibrillators (AICDs)

Automatic implantable defibrillators (AICDs) are very sophisticated devices that monitor and shock (defibrillate) the heart if a life threatening arrhythmia occurs. They are used in the prevention of sudden cardiac death, a condition caused from ventricular tachycardia and/or ventricular fibrillation.

Prior to the development of AICDs, the only treatment for patients at risk for this condition was antiarrhythmic medications. When compared to medical management with antiarrhythmic medications, AICDs are far superior at saving lives.

AICDs are two or three times larger than a pacemaker and are implanted in either the abdomen or the chest wall. The leads are much more sophisticated than those of a pacemaker as they have to be able to monitor the heart as well as deliver an effective shock when needed.

The surgery required to implant an AICD is more involved than pacemaker implantation. Whereas many cardiologists implant pacemakers, only cardiologists who specialize in the field of electrophysiology implant AICDs.

The devices can cost the hospital as much as $25,000 per unit. The cardiologist's fee for implantation approaches $2,000. In addition to these costs, the hospital charges for the use of the catheterization lab and post implantation monitoring. Keep in mind that these devices are only implanted if it is determined that the patient is at high risk for sudden cardiac death. Despite the expense involved in implanting AICDs the devices are one of the most cost effective therapies in cardiology because they are so effective at saving lives.

Newer AICDs double as pacemakers. When life-threatening rhythms first appear, such as ventricular tachycardia, the AICD will first attempt to "pace" the heart back to a regular rhythm before reverting to cardioversion (shock). This saves battery life and is much more comfortable, usually not even perceived by the patient.

6. Arrhythmias During Pregnancy

Cardiac rhythm disorders may occur during pregnancy in otherwise healthy women or as a consequence of underlying organic heart disease. Early recognition and appropriate intervention is important to reduce the potential of fetal and maternal injury.

Sustained arrhythmias occur at a frequency of one in 2000 pregnancies and the vast majority are supraventricular in origin. The exact incidence of transient nonsustained arrhythmic events is unknown, but these occur at a much higher frequency.

Several explanations for the increased incidence of arrhythmia during pregnancy are available. Blood volume increases significantly during pregnancy. A 30 to 40% increase above nonpregnant values is generally observed. This increase in blood volume leads to an increase in venous return to the heart and consequent swelling and stretching of the heart. In addition, the complex hormonal and autonomic changes during pregnancy may be implicated in the development of arrhythmia.

The therapy of arrhythmia during pregnancy presents several challenges. The physiologic changes during pregnancy may alter the pharmacokinetics of many drugs and thus influence side effect profiles and therapeutic responses. In addition, special attention should be given to the effects of drug therapy on the developing fetus and the possibility of passing the drug to the baby through breast milk after delivery.

The clinical presentation and diagnostic assessment of a pregnant patient with cardiac arrhythmias is similar to non-pregnant patients. These individuals may present with palpitations, dizziness, lightheadedness, syncope, shortness of breath or even overt heart failure. A detailed history and physical examination are most important to successful diagnosis. Careful attention should be directed at the possibility of any underlying heart disease. A baseline 12 lead electrocardiogram should be obtained in all patients. Some type of ambulatory electrocardiography is usually helpful. If the patient reports daily symptoms, than a 24 hour monitor is appropriate. However, if symptoms are more sporadic, then a 30 day event monitor will be more useful. A concurrent and careful diary kept by the patient is also very important in arriving at the correct diagnosis. Two-dimensional and Doppler echocardiography may be required in selected patients to assess cardiac function and anatomy.

Supraventricular Arrhythmias

Premature atrial beats are common during normal pregnancy. These arrhythmias are benign and do not require specific therapy beyond reassurance. Removal of caffeine, tobacco, alcohol or other stimulant substances is generally effective.

The incidence of supraventricular tachycardia during pregnancy has been estimated to be 2.6%. This estimate includes all types of tachycardia which are supraventricular in origin. Of these cases, atrial fibrillation is relatively uncommon occurring almost exclusively in the setting of rheumatic heart disease. True PSVT (paroxysmal supraventricular tachycardia) due to an extra electrical pathway in the heart, accounts for most of these problems during pregnancy. Although these patients are born with this problem, it is not unusual to present with the first episode of rapid heart rate during the first pregnancy. After delivery the rapid heart rate continues to be a problem for most patients and should be treated with medication or catheter ablation.

Nancy W. is a 28-year-old female in our practice who presented at 12 weeks of pregnancy with several new episodes of rapid heart rate that lasted up to 30 minutes. These episodes came on for no reason and terminated after lying down and deep breathing. These episodes caused profound dizziness and lightheadedness but no actual fainting. Based upon her history we diagnosed PSVT and treated her with a medication known to be safe during pregnancy (sotalol). After delivery of a healthy baby boy she continued to have problems with rapid heart rate and she underwent curative catheter ablation. The whole procedure took less than one hour. Catheter ablation is a safe, simple, nonsurgical, catheter based therapy that is performed on an outpatient basis and offers cure rates above 99%. No stitches or incisions are required. Because x-rays are necessary the procedure is not safe during pregnancy but can be performed shortly after delivery. Major complications are distinctly uncommon. Overall cure rates with the ablation approach for PSVT at the Orange County Heart Institute since 1994 have been 99.8%. Recurrences in the first year requiring a second procedure have been less than three percent and no major complications have occurred. Based upon our favorable experience with ablation, this therapy is recommended in most cases of PSVT.

Ventricular Arrhythmias

Premature ventricular beats (complexes) also frequently called PVCs are equally common during pregnancy. These patients are most frequently asymptomatic and require no therapy. In patients with symptoms of palpitations, skipped beats or dizziness, reassurance or removal of stimulants is generally effective. In patients with underlying structural heart disease and more complex arrhythmias, a signal averaged electrocardiogram should be considered. Ventricular tachycardia is defined as three or more successive beats of ventricular origin. Sustained ventricular tachycardia is characterized by instability or duration greater than 30 seconds and is generally quite symptomatic. Ventricular tachycardia is uncommon during pregnancy, occurring almost exclusively in the setting of serious underlying heart disease. Unstable arrhythmias including ventricular tachycardia should be treated with electricity in the form of direct current cardioversion. Stable arrhythmias can be treated with medication. Pregnant patients with sustained ventricular arrhythmias will often need to be hospitalized and should be on strict bed rest for most of their term.

Bradyarrhythmias

Bradycardia or slow heart rate may be due to sinus node dysfunction, wandering pacemaker or atrioventricular block; however, significant bradycardia during pregnancy is rare. Sinus bradycardia may occur on a transient basis and requires no therapy if asymptomatic. First degree and second degree atrioventricular block are also generally asymptomatic and seldom require therapy.

Symptomatic bradycardia during pregnancy is generally due to complete heart block or sick sinus syndrome. The treatment of symptomatic bradycardia is permanent pacemaker implantation. Acute management with temporary pacing, atropine or isuprel has also been utilized with no major morbidity. If possible, permanent pacemaker implantation should be delayed until the third trimester to protect the fetus from x-ray radiation exposure. In any case, optimal lead shielding of the fetus should be provided during any x-ray imaging for permanent pacemaker implantation Pregnancy in patients with permanent pacemakers is safe and well tolerated.

Specific Antiarrhythmic Therapy

The Food and Drug Agency (FDA) has categorized drugs according to their safety for use during pregnancy into Categories A, B, C, and D. Category A means the drugs have been prospectively tested in pregnant women and are safe. Unfortunately no category A drugs exist as pregnant women will not agree to any such studies. Category B means the drugs have been prospectively tested in pregnant animals and considerable clinical experience exists in pregnant women and the drugs appear safe. Category B drugs are the safest drugs available. Category C means that no testing has occurred but considerable clinical experience in pregnant women suggests the drugs are safe. Most drugs used in pregnancy are Category C. Category D drugs are not safe for use in pregnancy.

Sotalol is an antiarrhythmic medication available as a category B agent for use in pregnancy. It is excellent in maintaining normal sinus rhythm after cardioversion from atrial fibrillation and also has efficacy in the management of paroxysmal supraventricular tachycardia and ventricular arrhythmias.

Some beta blockers and acebutolol are also available as category B antiarrhythmic agents. These agents are most useful to control the ventricular response in atrial fibrillation; however, they also are useful in preventing paroxysmal supraventricular tachycardia episodes. All beta blockers can be used to prevent PAC's and PVC's and acebutolol is particularly useful in this type of arrhythmia.

Digoxin is useful in controlling the ventricular response during atrial fibrillation and in terminating or preventing paroxysmal supraventricular tachycardia episodes. Digoxin is a category C drug for use in pregnancy and it can cross the placenta. Adverse effects such as miscarriage during pregnancy have been reported if the mother becomes digoxin toxic. However, an extensive antenatal experience with digoxin has shown no evidence of birth defects and these agents are considered safe during pregnancy.

Other antiarrhythmic agents such as quinidine, procainamide and dissopyramide have efficacy in maintaining normal sinus rhythm after cardioversion from atrial fibrillation and in preventing sustained and nonsustained ventricular arrhythmias. Quinidine enjoys an extensive experience in the obstetric population, having been utilized since the 1930's. No formal trials of quinidine have been performed during pregnancy. However, the extensive use of this agent in pregnant women has not been associated with either birth defects or adverse fetal or maternal outcomes. All three agents are available as category C drugs for use in pregnancy.

Most arrhythmias occurring during pregnancy are benign and do not require specific antiarrhythmic therapy. Patient reassurance, anxiety controls and removal of exogenous stimulant substances is usually sufficient. Specific antiarrhythmic therapy for sustained or symptomatic nonsustained arrhythmias should be considered after carefully assessing the risk-benefit ratio. The most common sustained arrhythmia occurring during pregnancy is paroxysmal supraventricular tachycardia. In patients of child-bearing capacity with a history of sustained paroxysmal supraventricular tachycardia, counseling and education should be provided prior to pregnancy. Because pregnancy is likely to increase paroxysmal supraventricular tachycardia episodes, curative radiofrequency ablation should be strongly considered prior to conception.

Fetal birth defects due to drug exposure depend upon the drug involved, the length of drug exposure, the ability of the drug to cross the placenta and the genetic susceptibility of the fetus. Defects are most likely to occur during the first trimester of pregnancy. Therefore, whenever possible, antiarrhythmic drug therapy should be delayed until after the first trimester.

A Word About Magnesium Supplements

Magnesium is a mineral that helps regulate many bodily functions and the contraction of muscles and the conduction of nerve impulses. It is an often underused treatment for irregular heart beats. Many people, especially women, have palpitations that are very bothersome but not dangerous. These are usually due to extra or premature heart beats from the top or bottom chambers. If your doctor determines that you have benign PACs or PVCs, magnesium is a very effective and safe regimen. Magnesium also helps reduce the frequency of attacks of paroxysmal atrial fibrillation and supraventricular tachycardias.

The only caveat is that if you have kidney problems, magnesium should be used with caution, since it is excreted through the kidneys, and could build up to high levels. Even during pregnancy, when palpitations are particularly common, magnesium is safe and effective. Of course, do not take it without the approval of your doctor.

In summary, arrhythmias are common problems, especially in women. Palpitations, dizzy spells or fainting should be thoroughly evaluated by a cardiologist. Although arrhythmia can be life threatening, it can be accurately characterized with modern diagnostic techniques and then treated appropriately.

10

Diet and Heart Disease

Fast Fact
Every known diet that promotes weight loss depends on burning more calories than you consume. There is no variation of diet (low fat, low carbohydrate or high protein) that works through any other method than calories in versus calories out!

Myths, tips and the truth about what really works

Many people struggle with excess body weight or obesity for most of their lives. The weight loss industry is always emerging with the next "miracle weight loss diet" because the ability to maintain weight loss is so difficult. The high failure rate leaves the frustrated dieter always looking for, and willing to engage in, the latest fad. Many weight loss programs can be healthy, however, many are not. All require some degree of willpower. The closer the diet simulates your own personal taste, the more likely you'll succeed. However, if your personal taste inclines toward unhealthy foods, you may succeed in losing weight but fail at protecting your heart.

Here's the bottom line on weight reduction diets:

1. Every single diet that promotes weight loss depends on burning up more calories than you consume. It doesn't matter if it is a high fat diet, a high carbohydrate diet or something in between. Burning an excess of 3,500 calories more than you consume will add up to losing one pound of fat.

2. Most diets seem to work in the short term simply because a person is attentive to what they are eating, which results in less calorie consumption.

3. No combinations of foods will work together in some unique way to make you burn up more calories.

4. More frequent meals may help with weight loss. Your metabolism is increased throughout the day while your body burns calories digesting the food. So five or six meals may promote more weight loss than two or three meals per day with the same total number of calories.

5. There is no truth to the idea that eating your last meal before seven or eight at night will burn more calories through a change in metabolism. Those who try not to eat later in the evening generally can lose weight because they avoid the extra calories associated with late night snacking.

6. All diets that severely restrict carbohydrates, like the Atkins Diet or "liquid protein diets," produce a state of *ketosis*. Excess water loss and muscle loss occur. Your body requires carbohydrates to help metabolize fats. When fats are not completely metabolized, ketones are the result. Ketones cause a decrease in a sensation of hunger and also promote the excretion of excess water from the body. A lot of the initial and rapid weight loss is from water. The water will be retained as soon as any carbohydrates are consumed. The state of ketosis also promotes breakdown of your muscle mass. So after the water loss, a large proportion of the weight loss is from muscle and not just fat. Therefore, this approach is not healthy in the *long run* as a sustained diet.

7. Chromium supplements do not promote weight loss. Chromium is required for the secretion, production and use of insulin by our bodies. There is no evidence that it promotes weight loss.

8. Pyruvate is a supplement often promoted for weight loss. It is a naturally occurring metabolite of the energy producing cycles of all the cells of your body. It has not been proven to speed up the metabolism or promote weight loss.

9. Calcium consumed in dairy products or supplements seems to promote weight loss. How this mechanism may work is not clear.

10. You want to adopt a lifestyle that will work for the long term. This means a diet that will not deprive you of any one food group and contains adequate calories to maintain muscle mass. If the diet promotes muscle loss, your metabolism goes down and your ability to adequately exercise is greatly impaired. A calorie restricted diet without an increase or maintenance of exercise will result in your body reaching a new "set point." A "set point" means that your body decreases its metabolism in response to the reduced intake of calories. Your metabolism is therefore "reset" at a lower rate and you burn up fewer calories per day. So even though you take in fewer calories, your weight loss slows. The key is to exercise, plus reduce calories so your "set point" is the same and your metabolism remains high to promote continued weight loss. A combined approach, exercise *and* calorie restriction, will lead to sustained and healthy weight maintenance.

A word about fats

"Fat doesn't make you fat, carbohydrates make you fat." Is this the revolutionary mantra of Dr Atkins? No, this is the revolutionary argument put forth by Justus Liebig, a noted chemist and inventor of the bouillon cube and chemical fertilizers. His observation was based on the fact that few animal feeds contained fats and yet farmers were able fatten up livestock by feeding them low fat, high carbohydrate grain diets. He made this revolutionary statement 100 years before Dr. Atkins proclaimed his low carbohydrate, high fat diet program.

It is common knowledge now that not all fats in our diet are the same. There are "good fats" that can actually protect your heart and to some degree help with weight loss. There are "bad fats" that are bad for your heart and actually are stored differently in your body and have a higher tendency to add to body fat.

The Good Fats

Oils that contain monounsaturated, unsaturated fats, and polyunsaturated fatty acids can reduce total cholesterol and increase HDL cholesterol levels. The essential fatty acids, which the body can't make, include omega-3 (mainly from marine animals) and omega-6 fatty acids (from plant and animal sources). Unsaturated vegetable oils from canola, peanuts, olive, flax, corn, safflower and sunflower are heart healthy. Remember however, that if these oils are made into a softer margarine by a process called hydrogenation, they lose many of their health benefits and can actually become harmful. They are referred to as *trans fatty acids.*

The Bad Fats

Trans fatty acids
There is no question that trans fatty acids have a deleterious effect on cholesterol levels and increase the risk of heart disease. They increase total cholesterol levels and LDL cholesterol levels, and reduce HDL cholesterol levels. They are also contributors to inflammation of the lining of the arteries. There is a major push in the food industry to eliminate transfats from the cooking process by developing new types of healthy fats for cooking. Manufacturers began substituting partially hydrogenated vegetable oils for saturated fats in processed foods as a way of making the fats healthier and less likely to spoil, only to find out that these transfats were a major contributor to heart disease. Foods that contain relatively large amounts of trans fatty acids are high-fat baked goods, especially doughnuts, cookies, french fries, potato chips, corn chips and many crackers and cakes. Also note any product whose label says "partially hydrogenated vegetable oils," virtually all processed foods, and margarines. The more solid the margarine, the more the trans fatty acids. As of 2006,

the FDA requires labeling of food for trans fatty acid content. There is no level of trans fatty acids regarded as safe.

Saturated fats

Saturated fatty acids come from animal fats (meat, dairy products, lard) as well as tropical oils such as coconut and palm oils. They raise the levels of LDL cholesterol. It has been known for many decades that these types of fats were not heart healthy. This led to the switch to unsaturated fats, vegetable oils, by the food manufacturers. However, food made from unsaturated fats readily became rancid. In a search to stabilize and add shelf life to the food, a hydrogen atom was added to the fat, which made the vegetable oil more solid and gave it a longer shelf life. These *partially hydrogenated oils,* though of vegetable origin, are unhealthy for our hearts.

A word about carbohydrates

Carbohydrates are an essential form of energy. They are best described in terms of their ability to raise blood sugar. Those that raise blood sugar quickly, like white bread, are considered high glycemic (glycemic means blood sugar), and less beneficial to your health. Darker or colored foods, like vegetables and brown rice, are considered low glycemic because they raise blood sugar to a lesser degree, or less quickly and so are considered more healthful.

A word about protein

Protein is essential to maintaining muscle mass and strength. Many people assume that only meat can provide protein of good quality. Actually, egg whites and whey from milk are the near perfect protein. Many vegetables can provide excellent sources of protein if meats are not desired. Many cultures live on fish without any other animal protein and maintain excellent health.

Comparing Diets

Is there a diet that helps maintain weight *and* protects your heart? Are low carbohydrates the best way to go? Is the ultra-low fat diet the best protection for your heart?

The simplest way to come up with the proper diet is to think of what you want from the diet. You want to maintain physical conditioning to live an active life. You want a diet that will not inflame the coronary arteries or promote plaque buildup. You want a diet that will maintain a healthy and proper body weight.

Low carbohydrate, moderate protein diets (Atkins, South Beach)

Carbohydrates create the main fuel for exercising muscles. If carbohydrates are restricted, there is fatigue, and muscles are broken down to be used as fuel. Carbohydrates are needed to promote protein uptake by the muscles to be used for repair and rebuilding of the muscle. Without carbohydrates, your muscles waste because they are cannibalized for fuel, and they do not have the protein available to them for repair. Not a good long term diet if you believe that exercise is crucial for your heart; not a good long term diet that will allow you to maintain your muscle mass so you can exercise, work or do daily household chores. Initial weight loss is from fluid loss due to ketosis, which occurs from incomplete metabolism of fats when adequate carbohydrates are not available. The Atkins Diet allows high amounts of saturated fats. It will promote weight loss but many people develop a "diet drift," which means as time goes on, they increase their carbohydrate intake plus maintain a high fat diet. Bottom line: not a good long term diet.

The South Beach Diet is more reasonable. The carbohydrate restriction emphasizes low glycemic carbohydrates, those that do not cause a rapid increase in blood sugar which promotes fat formation. The fats in the South Beach Diet tend to be the healthier mono and polyunsaturated fats.

Low carbohydrate, high protein, moderate fat (Scarsdale Diet, Zone Diet)

The basic tenet of these diets is that high carbohydrate consumption leads to weight gain. The Zone Diet requires exact ratios to balance each other: 40% carbs, 30% protein and 30% fat. The carbohydrates release insulin which decrease blood sugar levels and promote fat storage, but the protein releases the hormone glucagon which stimulates carbohydrate release from the liver and raises blood sugar. The fats ingested release hormones that regulate the release of fat from cells. A balance occurs that promotes weight loss. The Scarsdale Diet dictates 34.5% carbs, 43% protein, 22.5% fat, and a 1,000 calorie a day diet for two weeks, after which calories increase.

Results of these diets are similar to those from Atkins: problems of fatigue and muscle wasting and initial large weight loss from water loss.

High carbohydrate, moderate protein, extreme low fat diet (Pritikin, Ornish)

Fats are required for fuel for bursts of muscle activity, like lifting and sprinting. Good fats (monosaturated and polyunsaturated fats) are needed for cell function; they have anti-inflammatory properties and stabilize heart rhythms. Bad fats (saturated fats found in meats and transfats found in snacks, crackers, etc.) can inflame the lining of the coronary arteries when taken in large quantities. Extremely low fat diets (less than 10% fat) have in a few limited studies shown to reverse or slow the build up of plaque. The Pritikin approach is eating foods that are not calorie dense, that is, they have less than 400 calories per pound, like vegetables, and a small amount of meat and dairy products. The Ornish approach is very restricted in fats, including healthy fats in nuts and monosaturated oils, like canola and olive oil. Extremely low fat diets are difficult to live with. The low fats can lead to nutrient deficiencies, a drop in HDL and an increase in triglycerides. In addition, the high carbohydrate intake promotes insulin resistance and is therefore not good for diabetics.

It should be noted that moderately low fat diets (25 to 30% fat) have also been shown to slow or reverse the buildup of plaque. Moderately low fat diets are easily adapted to most life styles and are enjoyable and sustainable for life.

Moderate carbohydrate (50 to 60%), moderate protein (15 to 30%), low fat (25 to 40%) (Mediterranean diet, The OC Cure For Heart Disease, Andrew Weil Diet, US Food Pyramid, Weight Watchers)

There is ample evidence of the benefit of a Mediterranean diet that has as its cornerstone healthy monosaturated fats, large quantities of vegetables, legumes and modest carbohydrates. All of the above diets revolve more or less around those principles. Some emphasize low glycemic carbohydrates and more exact ratios of macronutrients (OC Cure For Heart Disease or Andrew Weil Diet) and lower fats. The mainstay of nutritional thinking is that all the macronutrients (macronutrients are carbs, protein and fat; micronutrients are vitamin and minerals) are important for general health, and the extreme exclusion of any one group is not only unhealthy but also unsustainable for a lifestyle. Low glycemic carbohydrates are carbs that are slowly absorbed by the intestine. They do not cause drastic increases in insulin spikes with a subsequent drop in blood sugar and resultant hunger and fatigue. There is also more and more evidence that low glycemic diets help raise HDL cholesterol (the good cholesterol), lower triglycerides, and more importantly fight inflammation of the coronary arteries since they lower C-reactive protein (CRP), which is a marker of inflammation.

So, how do we put all the confusing data in perspective? Two recent studies revealed the following:

1. *Comparison of the Atkins, Ornish, Weight Watchers, and Zone diets for weight loss and heart disease risk reduction: a randomized trial.*

This study compared these diets over a year and failed to show any significant differences in weight loss. More people were able to stick to the Zone and Weight Watchers than to the Atkins and Ornish diets, probably due to the more extreme nature of the latter two.

2. The Nurses Health Study: Low-Carbohydrate-Diet Score and the Risk of Coronary Heart Disease in Women

This study reviewed the record of 83,000 women followed over two decades in the on-going Nurses Health Study. It was found that (1) lots of calories from refined sugars (high glycemic carbs) and highly processed foods (high saturated fats) nearly doubled the risk of heart disease; and (2) those on low carbohydrate diets with protein and fat sources from vegetables rather than animal sources (that is, more mono and unsaturated fats), had 30% less heart disease.

*The findings suggest that diets lower in carbohydrate and higher in protein and fat are **not** associated with increased risk of coronary heart disease in women.* When vegetable sources of fat and protein are chosen, these diets may moderately reduce the risk of coronary heart disease.

The Bottom Line

1. For the best chance of long term success, choose a diet that does not exclude food groups that you naturally enjoy. For instance, if you tend to enjoy bread and pastas, a low carb diet will not be sustainable.

2. Low carb diets tend to help lower triglycerides and raise HDL cholesterol, whereas, low fat diets were better in lowering high LDL cholesterol levels. Choosing a diet based on your lipid profile may be reasonable for some people. Choosing a diet that is palatable results in a higher likelihood of long term adherence.

3. Weight loss will occur when calories burned are more than calories consumed, regardless of the diet. The large initial weight loss with low carb diets is mainly water.

4. *Carbohydrate restriction will not increase the risk of heart disease. Moderate carbohydrate diet with low glycemic type of carbs may lower your risk of heart disease.* Moderate to high carbohydrate diets with high glycemic carbs can increase your risk of heart disease. Carbohydrates are essential for strength training, which along with aerobic exercise is crucial for maximum heart health and well being.

5. Moderate low-fat diets that emphasize monosaturated fats (olive oil and canola oil), and omega 3 fatty acids (cold water fatty fish like salmon, herring and sardines), and plant sources (nuts, flaxseed and avocado) are the most heart healthy diets.

6. Protein sources in moderation, 15 to 30% of calories; sometimes more if bodybuilding is desired (about one gram of protein per kilogram of body weight per day) are all reasonable and scientifically backed approaches to a heart healthy diet.

7. A Mediterranean diet, and the diet proposed in *The OC Cure for Heart Disease, (co-authored by Dr. Lawrence Santora, Dick Butkus and Dr. Steve Armentrout),* tend best to meet the criteria for a diet that is sustainable, heart healthy and adaptable to weight loss, while maintaining muscle mass and quality of life.

11

Vitamins and Supplements

The world of vitamins and supplements is forever changing. What was hot a few years ago may this year be considered harmful to your health, or at least not helpful. The truth is, few supplements have strong scientific bases upon which to recommend their use to promote heart health. Despite this lack of proof, many people still want to take vitamins and supplements if they believe they feel better taking them, or if there is even a slim chance the supplement may be at least a little bit helpful.

Supplements

Aspirin

Aspirin is without question beneficial in preventing a second heart attack or a second stroke in both men and women. However, recently completed studies in women under age 65 without known heart disease revealed that daily aspirin did not cause a reduction in their chance of a heart attack compared to the same aged women who took a placebo. Aspirin did cause a reduction in the chance of a first stroke in women.

Final word: If you are under 65, and you have coronary calcium on an EBCT heart scan, low dose aspirin would be beneficial in preventing a heart attack and stroke. Most women over 65 benefit from low dose aspirin even if there is no coronary calcium.

Calcium

Calcium supplements seem to have no particular benefits for the heart in women who are otherwise healthy. Calcium taken in food has nothing to do with the calcium in the plaque that forms in the coronary arteries. If you do have an EBCT coronary calcium scan, and calcium (plaque) is identified, you do not have to modify your calcium intake. Likewise, calcium in food will not interfere with the function of certain blood pressure medications referred to as "calcium channel blockers."

Final word: Calcium supplements are not needed for heart protection.

Coenzyme Q10

CoQ10 may have benefits in reducing muscle aches in those taking statins. There is some evidence that it may help some patients with congestive heart failure.

Final word: CoQ10, about 50 mg per day for those with mild muscle cramps taking statins. Much higher doses, about 200 mg per day, may help some patients with congestive heart failure, under the direction of their doctor, of course.

Cholestin

Cholestin is a weak form of a statin made from red rice yeast. It is the same ingredient in Mevacor (lovastatin), but the potency and consistency is less than commercial lovastatin.

Final word: Cholestin will lower cholesterol to a slight degree. If significant lowering of cholesterol is needed, commercial statins are probably more effective.

Garlic

Garlic has anti-oxidant, anticlotting and cholesterol lowering properties. There is some evidence that garlic lowers blood pressure and homocysteine levels. Aged garlic seems to be the most effective. Some supplements are odor free. High doses may increase the risk of bleeding in those taking blood thinners like warfarin.

Final word: A clove or more of garlic per day may have some benefit in lowering cholesterol and blood pressure.

Guggalgum (Gugulipid)

Weakly lowers cholesterol.

Final word: About 75 mgs per day may be helpful for those who cannot tolerate commercially available cholesterol medications.

Hawthorn

Hawthorn dilates the arteries and weakly lowers blood pressure in a method similar to the commonly used ACE inhibitor blood pressure medications. There is weak evidence that it may help patients with congestive heart failure.

Final word: Hawthorne may help as an adjunct to the usual treatments for congestive heart failure, under the guidance of a doctor. Effective dose is unknown.

Policosanol

Policosanol lowers cholesterol by inhibiting its production. It is made from rice-bran wax or sugar cane. The studies showing that ploicosanol lowers cholesterol have been criticized as not scientifically rigorous.

Final word: Ten to twenty mgs per day may be helpful.

Functional foods

Milk fortified with omega 3 fatty acids

An as yet undeveloped but ingenious new functional would be to combine the protein and other nutritional benefits of milk with outstanding heart benefits of omega 3 fatty acids. The combination of fish oil with non fat milk without altering the taste of the milk may be one of the best food products available when developed.

Final word: One or more eight ounce glasses per day, when available.

Soy protein

Soy protein can lower total and LDL cholesterol about 10% and comes in many forms including powders, nuts and other processed foods.

Final word: Usually about 20 to 25 gms of soy protein per day, the equivalent to about two and one-half cups of soy milk, is the effective amount.

Margarines that lower cholesterol

Benecol and Take Control are plant derived margarines that inhibit cholesterol absorption in the intestine.

Final word: A one gm serving each day can result in about a seven percent LDL reduction.

Alcohol

One drink per day for women has shown benefit in protecting from heart disease. One drink is one ounce of alcohol, four ounces of wine or twelve ounces of beer. Men seem to benefit with up to two drinks per day.

Final word: Unless you enjoy alcohol, it is probably not worthwhile making it a part of your heart protection regimen. If you do, use no more than one drink a day.

Vitamins

Vitamin A (beta carotene)

Vitamin A is a known antioxidant when taken naturally in foods. However, when taken as a supplement no benefit is seen in preventing heart disease. Some evidence that smokers who took Vitamin A and continued to smoke, had a higher incidence of lung cancer than those who did not take Vitamin A.

Final word: Do not take Vitamin A or beta carotene with the thought of preventing heart disease.

Vitamin C

Vitamin C has no conclusive benefit in preventing heart disease. One study showed an adverse reaction in patients taking statins (cholesterol lowering drugs) plus Vitamin C and E. Those taking a statin and Vitamin C and E had more heart attacks than those taking the statin alone.

Final word: Limit Vitamin C to 500 mg or less per day unless your doctor recommends higher doses for other non heart related benefits.

Vitamin E

Vitamin E produced a similar outcome as Vitamin C when combined with statins in the heart protection study mentioned earlier.

Final word: Limit the dose of Vitamin E to 400 iu per day, unless your doctor recommends higher doses for other non heart related benefits.

Vitamin B3 (niacin)

Niacin is one of the most important vitamins for heart health. However, the dose needed is at least 500 mg per day; much higher than the 30 to 50 mg found in most multivitamins. A common dose is 500 mg to 1000 mg per day, often up to 3000 mg per day. These doses can cause possible liver inflammation, and therefore require physician supervision.

Niacin is the most effective medication for raising HDL cholesterol. In addition, niacin enlarges the LDL cholesterol particle to the less dangerous larger size. It is also very effective in lowering the triglyceride levels and the levels of the potentially dangerous lipoprotein (a) [Lp(a)]. Niacin is often used as a complement to statin medications, since niacin modifies many of the lipid problems not touched by statin medications. Note that "flush free" niacin varieties are the least effective type in lowering cholesterol.

Final word: Niacin is one of the most important vitamins for heart health when used under the direction of a doctor.

Vitamin B6 (pyridoxine)

A dose of 50 mg per day of pyridoxine is effective for high homocysteine levels. Pyridoxine has been shown to reduce the chance of arteries re-narrowing after PTCA when combined with folic acid and Vitamin B12. These three B vitamins all help reduce homocysteine levels.

Final word: Pyridoxine at 50 mg a day may be a beneficial supplement for heart protection. Doses should never be more than 200 mg per day because of possible nerve toxicity.

Vitamin B12

Vitamin B12 has a complementary effect with folic acid and pyridoxine in treating high homocysteine levels.

Final word: A dose of 1000 micrograms per day is reasonable for high homocysteine levels.

Folic acid

Folic acid has a complementary effect on lowering homocysteine levels with the other B vitamins.

Final word: A dose of 400 mcg to 1000 mcg per day of folic acid is reasonable as a daily supplement. Almost all multivitamins have 400 mcg of folic acid. To treat high homocysteine levels, 1000 to 2500 ug per day are needed.

Final recommendations: If you have coronary calcium on an EBCT scan, taking 81 mg of aspirin, 2,000 to 6,000 mg of fish oil caps, 50 mg of pyridoxine (B$_6$), 1,000 ug of B$_{12}$, and 400 iu of folic acid are reasonable, plus whatever cholesterol modifying medications are recommended by your doctor. If you have never had an EBCT calcium scan, have never been known to have heart disease and have a normal cholesterol profile, it would be reasonable to take a multivitamin and fish oil capsules totaling about 2,000 mg per day. Remember, however, there are no scientific studies that show vitamins have any strong benefit in preventing heart disease.

12

Hormone Replacement Therapy

It has been a long journey for hormone replacement therapy, from its rise in popularity in the early 1960s to its recent precipitous fall. An overview will give you a better understanding of how medical thinking is affected at times and will help you to have a better grasp of what is available.

In 1966, a New York gynecologist named Robert Wilson, MD, wrote a best seller, *Feminine Forever.* In his book, menopause was promoted as a condition of "living decay." Menopause was portrayed as a tragedy for a woman "which often destroys her character as well as her health." Estrogen was to be a rejuvenator for a woman to help her to be "...much more pleasant to live with and not become dull and unattractive." The book became a sensation and the hormone's chief manufacturer, Wyeth Pharmaceuticals, advanced the success of estrogen. An ad in 1975 read: "Almost any tranquilizer might calm her down...but at her age, estrogen may be what she really needs." These concepts all went forward even though the FDA refuted Dr. Wilson's claims as unsubstantiated. For the next two decades estrogen was the drug of choice to salvage one's beauty and health.

In 1975, *The New England Journal of Medicine* published an article in which it was shown that there was an increased risk of uterine cancer with the use of estrogen. Later on, the combination therapy of estrogen and progestin was introduced to have a protective effect in those women with an intact uterus. This finding did not deter the push towards hormone replacement therapy since some epidemiologic studies were showing possible protection from heart disease in women taking the hormone therapy. However, these studies were not the "gold standard" research in medicine since they did not look for cause and effect, but only trend and possible relation.

By 1990, hormone therapy was the expected treatment for post menopausal women. If a woman was not on the medication, she would be referred to her gynecologist to insure that she was treated appropriately and protected from heart disease.

However, about this time, clinical trials were coming out with surprising results. Clinical studies are considered the "gold standard" for providing cause and effect relationships between a disease process and a proposed treatment. "Postmenopausal Estrogen/Progestin Interventions Trial" or PEPI, began in 1987. The National Heart, Lung, and Blood Institute (NHLB) and some other units of the National Institutes of Health (NIH) supported PEPI. It looked at the effects of different hormone therapy regimens on predominantly white healthy women between the ages of 45 and 64. The study took three years, followed 875 women and showed that "bad" LDL cholesterol was reduced and "good" HDL cholesterol was increased with either estrogen alone or in combination with progestin. It also revealed that a large percentage of those who took estrogen alone developed an overgrowth of the lining of their uterus. This finding prompted the caution for women who still had their uteruses to take estrogen with progestin.

The study that started the change in our thinking about hormone replacement therapy, (and itself somewhat controversial), was "Heart and Estrogen-Progestin Replacement Study" or HERS. Enrollment started in 1983 and the study looked at whether the combination therapy of estrogen and progestin protected women with heart disease from a second heart attack. Average age of these 2,763 women was 67. The results of the study, released in the *Journal of the American Medical Association*, was a shock to the pharmaceutical company, Wyeth, which had supported the study in hopes of consolidating the claim that this combination medication was heart-protective. Results showed that the hormone therapy not only did *not* protect women from another heart attack, but actually increased their risk for another heart attack during the first year of the therapy. The study also showed an increase in the risk of blood clots in the lungs and legs.

The study was criticized based on the average age of the patients; there was also the thought that a longer follow-up might show some protection from further heart attacks. Therefore, some of the patients were followed for another two and a half years, during which time no benefit was observed. The medical community had to consider that up to the release of the results of the two trials, our support for estrogen and progestin in protecting against heart disease was based only on observational and anecdotal findings.

The conclusions of the studies were that hormone combination therapy should not be given as a protective agent against future heart attacks in women with known heart disease. This kind of therapy (which is called a secondary therapy) was not recommended. We need to realize that the combination therapy in all the trials has been with the current conventional one called Prempro with dosing of estrogen (0.625 mg) and progestin (2.5 mg).

While the medical society and patients were dealing with these findings and the change in the perception of the effects of hormone therapy, the "Women's Health Initiative," or WHI, was underway. This study, supported by the NHLB, included 161,000 healthy, postmenopausal women. It was initiated in 1991, is one of the largest studies ever in the United States, and includes several trials. The postmenopausal hormone therapy clinical trial, whose goal was to see if hormone therapy protected against heart disease and hip fracture, had two arms, one looking at the combination of estrogen and progestin and the other at estrogen alone. The drug was compared to a placebo (a sugar pill) in each arm. Over 16,000 women took the combination therapy or a placebo, another 10,739 women who did not have a uterus took either the estrogen alone or a placebo. The study was supposed to end in 2005; however, the combination therapy arm of the study was stopped early in July 2002 because the safety board found that there was an increased risk of breast cancer. It also found that the overall risks of taking these hormones outnumbered the benefits. There was increased risk for breast cancer, heart attacks, strokes and blood clots. The benefits were decreased risk for hip fracture and colon cancer.

The other arm of the trial was looking at estrogen alone and that one was stopped early in May 2004 when it did not show any benefit and an increased risk of stroke.

Based on the findings in July of 2002, the American Heart Association president at the time, Dr. Bonow, published this statement: "Based on current evidence, the American Heart Association advises that women do not start or continue combined HRT for the prevention of coronary heart disease."

The FDA also added a black box warning for the use of combination hormone therapy cautioning patients and physicians against the use for primary or secondary prevention purposes.

Where does this leave us? Each woman has to look at the benefits and risks of taking hormone therapy and talk to her physician. At this time, medical society is not recommending hormone therapy for treatment or protection against heart disease. However, estrogen is still the only medication that helps with menopausal symptoms. If you decide to take the medication for menopausal symptoms, then you should discuss it with your physician. At this time, it is recommended that use be limited to the shortest period for management of symptoms.

Fortunately, there are many ongoing studies looking into different doses and different routes of administering hormone therapy. The findings will help both the gynecologic and cardiac societies to better treat their patients.

Alternative Treatments

Many different treatments have been tried to alleviate the symptoms associated with menopause. However, estrogen still remains the most effective treatment.

Black Cohosh, ginseng, and St. John's Wort are among some of the popular over-the-counter herbal treatments. In clinical studies, none of these options did better than placebo, however, it should be noted that some people do feel better with these treatments despite the lack of scientific support.

Vitamin E has also been used as an alternative, but this vitamin is not recommended at doses above 400 iu/day because it has been shown to have a negative cardiovascular impact.

Phytoestrogens (soy), SSRI (selective serotonin receptive inhibitors) antidepressants, and clonidine, a blood pressure medication, are other types of alternative therapy. Again, when compared to placebo treatments, none of them have been superior to treat menopausal symptoms. However, there are some points to be emphasized. The SSRI antidepressants are helpful for menopausal patients with anxiety, depressive symptoms and sleep problems. Clonidine can be considered for menopausal patients with high blood pressure.

Finally, lifestyle changes can be tried. Wearing layered clothing, carrying a small fan and drinking plenty of water, are some of the recommendations that seem to help some patients.

Until we have more information, our recommendation is to use estrogen cautiously and for the shortest duration of time.

13

Exercise:
There Is No Substitute

No medication, vitamin or supplement provides the amazing array of health benefits that exercise affords. Your exercise program can be complex and regimented or the simplest form of walking. The scientific evidence is that any amount of exercise will benefit your heart directly, and indirectly, by improving all the known modifiable risk factors. Every age group can improve quality of life with exercise.

Benefits

- Reduces the tendency of blood to clot
- Reduces wide swings in adrenaline levels associated with stress
- Prevents osteoporosis
- Elevates mood
- Lowers blood pressure
- Helps control blood sugar, especially in diabetics
- Raises the good cholesterol (HDL cholesterol)
- Lowers the bad cholesterol (LDL cholesterol)
- Lowers triglycerides
- Promotes collateral blood vessel growth in coronary arteries
- Promotes long term weight loss
- Slows memory decline associated with the aging process
- Prolongs life expectancy

Types of exercise

1. Strength Training

Strength training was at one time an overlooked exercise for women. The popular thinking was that weight training was a man's exercise and large muscles were distinctly not feminine. However, it is clear that women just do not build large muscles due to their significantly lower testosterone levels. However, you can build strength. You can build muscle mass which helps burn more calories. And you can develop a slimmer body profile since muscle mass of the same weight occupies a smaller profile than fat. That is, you will lose inches but your weight may stay the same. The woman who engages in weight training will be less prone to injury since stronger muscles surrounding the joints will make the joint more stable. Though aerobic exercise prevents osteoporosis, strength training is superior in preventing fractures since bones need weight bearing stress to increase density.

Simplified Approach

Any type of simple device will work: water bottles, light dumbbells, soup cans or simple stretch bands. If you are on vacation, you can do single arm exercises with a small carry-on bag or even a purse that can be made heavier by placing water bottles or books inside.

How heavy?

Choose a weight you can lift 12 to 15 times without straining or holding your breath on the last repetition. This is "aerobic weight lifting" and is a good compromise to add strength, toning and muscle mass. Two sets of each exercise is a reasonable approach. If more muscle bulk is desired, increase the weight or resistance such that six to eight repetitions are the maximum you can do with that particular weight.

How frequently?

Two to three 30 minute sessions per week is reasonable. Unlike aerobic exercise, which should be done five to seven days per week, weight training requires that the muscles rest for a day or two in between sessions to allow muscle fibers to repair themselves.

What muscle groups?

Ideally all muscle groups should be exercised. Compound exercises are those that use multiple muscle groups at once and give the most health benefits for the least amount of time. Squats, push ups, lunges, pull ups and sit ups all contribute to building your core muscles, that is, the major muscles of the abdomen and back that maintain posture. For maximum benefit, do the large muscle groups first. For instance, exercise shoulder and chest muscles first, before exercising triceps and biceps.

2. Aerobic exercise

Any daily exercise is aerobic. It can be chasing kids around the house or vacuuming. There is a method to quantitate these chores for those who are too busy to walk on a regular basis or go to a gym. This method uses a pedometer and an aerobic mile equivalent chart. A total activity of five miles per day is a reasonable goal and can be added to the *10,000 Steps A Day Program* which follows. As a rule of thumb, you need about 10 to 15 aerobic miles per week to raise HDL, or 10,000 steps per day for at least six days per week.

The 10,000 Step Program is well proven and workable for any person, but especially for those women who have to divide their time between child care, household chores and career. For many, there is little time left for a personal workout. A simple pedometer will give feedback and benchmarks that can be used as guidelines to increase or maintain activity. Usual household chores, sedentary work and taking care of children add up to about three miles of aerobic activity, or about 6,000 steps. To gain additional health benefits of aerobic activity, like weight loss, raising HDL cholesterol and lowering blood pressure, a total of 10,000 steps per day is a reasonable goal. More than 10,000 steps will burn up more calories and cause additional weight loss.

Common sense activities will add the other 4,000 steps

per day: for instance, doing additional yard work, parking at the far end of the lot when shopping, or taking stairs instead of elevators. Set a goal to start of at least 10 miles per week.

Treadmill – Walking – Biking – Swimming

As a rough guideline, 30 minutes per day of any combination of these activities, six to seven days a week is recommended. The activity can be divided into 10 or 15 minute sessions with similar benefits. Keep in mind that the exercise you enjoy is the exercise that you will most likely stay with on a consistent basis. Also remember that any activity which needs the body to support its entire weight will burn more calories per hour. Therefore, swimming burns less calories per hour than biking since the water is supporting the body. Likewise, a walking exercise burns more calories than biking of similar intensity since part of the body weight is being supported on the bike.

Intensity of exercise

How do you measure the intensity of your exercise? The two simplest methods are the *target heart rate method* and the *rate of perceived exertion method.* The target heart rate method is attractive to many people since it gives a number that can easily be measured with inexpensive heart rate monitors.

Target heart rate method

The formula of 220 minus your age is used to determine your maximum heart rate. To then determine your target heart rate for fat burning, take 70 to 85% of your maximum heart rate. This will be the rate range to maintain during your walk.

Rate of perceived exertion or the "talk test"

Aerobic means "with oxygen." To burn the most fat, oxygen is needed. So the intensity of exercise should be high enough to increase the respiratory rate, but not so intense that your breathing cannot keep up with the exercise and becomes anaerobic, which means "without oxygen." Exercising to an intensity of "moderately strong" is the target intensity. This corresponds to

AEROBIC MILE EQUIVALENTS

Minutes of continous exercise
equal to a one mile run

	Easy	Moderate	Vigorous
Aerobic Dance	30	20	15
Backpacking	15	12	10
Basketball	20	12	10
Bicycling	18	14	10
(10, 14, & 18 mph pace)			
Calisthenics	18	15	15
Canoeing/Rowing	20	12	12
Cycling, stationary	16	11	11
(4, 6, 8 METS)			
Football	20	12	12
Gardening	60	30	30
Golfing	60	30	30
(Carrying Clubs/Pulling Cart)			
Hiking, Cross Country & Hills	20	12	12
Mountain Climbing	15	12	10
Racquetball, Handball, Squash	20	12	10
Rope Skipping	11	8	8
Running	12	8	8
SCUBA Diving	20	10	10
Skating	20	12	12
Skiing, Cross-Country	17	8	8
Skiing Downhill	60	20	20
Soccer	15	10	10
Stair or Bench Stepping	15	11	11
Swimming	18	11	11
Table Tennis	60	20	20
Tennis	20	11	11
Vollyeball	20	12	12
Walking	24	15	15
(24, 20, 15 min/mile pace)			
Water Skiing	30	15	15
Weight Training, Circuit	30	15	15

the "talk test": you are slightly to moderately short of breath, yet you can still carry on a conversation without hesitating between words. The nice thing about this method, as opposed to the target heart rate method, is that the "talk test" is not influenced by medications. Many blood pressure medications, like beta blockers and some calcium channel blockers, keep the heart rate lower than it normally would be. This naturally invalidates the target heart rate method but not the talk test method.

In summary, exercise is the cheapest and most effective method to prolong your life and improve its quality. Choose a method that suits your time constraints. Choose an exercise that you enjoy and start slowly. Get approval from your doctor before embarking on an exercise program, especially if you are over 40 years old and have any risk factors. You may benefit from a stress test before you start your exercise program. Start three to four days per week, work up to six to seven days per week. Add strength training two to three time per week. Stretch before each exercise session and drink plenty of fluids.

Addendum A
References

EBCT and CT angiography

1. Santora L, Marin J, Vangrow J, Minegar C, Robinson M, Mora J, Friede G. "Coronary Calcification in Anabolic Steroid Users." *Preventive Cardiology*, Fall 2006.

2. Budoff, Matthew J. MD; Shokooh, Shalizeh MD; Shavelle, Robert M. PhD; Kim, H. Tina MD; French, William J. MD, "Electron beam tomography and angiography: Sex differences." *American Heart Journal*. May 2002,143(5):877-882.

3. Arad Y, Spadaro LA, Roth M, Newstein D, Guerci AD. "Treatment of asymptomatic adults with elevated coronary calcium scores with atorvastatin, vitamin C, and vitamin E: the St. Francis Heart Study randomized clinical trial." *J Am Coll Cardiol*. 2005; 46:166–172.

4. Rasouli ML, Nasir K, Blumenthal RS, Park R, Aziz DC, Budoff MJ. "Plasma homocysteine predicts progression of atherosclerosis." *Atherosclerosis*. 2005 Jul; 181(1):159-65.

5. Taylor AJ, Bindeman J, Feuerstein I, Cao F, Brazaitis M, O'Malley PG. "Coronary calcium independently predicts incident premature coronary heart disease over measured cardiovascular risk factors: mean three-year outcomes in the Prospective Army Coronary Calcium (PACC) project."*J Am Coll Cardiol.* 2005 Sep 6; 46(5):807-14.

6. Arad Y, Goodman KJ, Roth M, Newstein D, Guerci AD. "Coronary calcification, coronary disease risk factors, C-reactive protein, and atherosclerotic cardiovascular disease events: the St. Francis Heart Study." *J Am Coll Cardiol.* 2005 Jul 5; 46(1):158-65.

7. Budoff MJ, Chen GP, Hunter CJ, Takasu J, Agrawal N, Sorochinsky B, Mao S. "Effects of hormone replacement on progression of coronary calcium as measured by electron beam tomography."*J Womens Health (Larchmt).* 2005 Jun;14(5):410-417. Addendum C References *237.*

8. LaMonte MJ, FitzGerald SJ, Church TS, Barlow CE, Radford NB, Levine BD, Pippin JJ, Gibbons LW, Blair SN, Nichaman MZ. "Coronary artery calcium score and coronary heart disease events in a large cohort of asymptomatic men and women." *Am J Epidemiol.* 2005 Sep 1;162(5):421-9.Epub 005 Aug 2.

9. Shemesh J, Koren-Morag N, Apter S, Rozenman J, Kirwan BA, Itzchak Y, Motro M. "Accelerated progression of coronary calcification: four-year follow-up in patients with stable coronary artery disease." *Radiology.* 2004 Oct; 233(1):201-Epub 2004 Aug 27.

10. Michos ED, Vasamreddy CR, Becker DM, Yanek LR, Moy TF, Fishman EK, Becker LC, Blumenthal RS. "Women with a low Framingham risk score and a family history of premature coronary heart disease have a high prevalence of subclinical coronary atherosclerosis." *Am Heart J.* 2005 Dec; 150(6):1276.

11. Khurana C, Rosenbaum CG, Howard BV, Adams-Campbell L, Detrano R, Klouj A, Hsia J. "Coronary Calcification in Black Women and White Women." *Am Heart J* 2003;145:724-729.

12. Hunold P, Vogt FM, Schmermund A, et al. "Radiation exposure during cardiac CT: effective doses at multi-detector row CT and electron-beam CT." *Radiology* 2003;226:145–52.

13. Morin RL, Gerber TC, McCollough CH. "Radiation dose in computed tomography of the heart." *Circulation* 2003;107:917–22.

14. Jakobs TF, Becker CR, Ohnesorge B, et al. "Multislice helical CT of the heart with retrospective ECG gating: reduction of radiation exposure by ECG-controlled tube current modulation." *Eur Radiol* 2002;12:1081–6.

15. Kuettner A, Beck T, Drosch T, et al. "Diagnostic accuracy of noninvasive coronary imaging using 16-detector slice spiral computed tomography with 188 ms temporal resolution." *J Am Coll Cardiol* 2005;45:123–7.

16. Mollet NR, Cademartiri F, Krestin GP, et al. "Improved diagnostic accuracy with 16-row multi-slice computed tomography coronary angiography." *J Am Coll Cardiol* 2005;45:128 –32.

17. Cerqueira MD, Weissman NJ, Dilsizian V, et al. "Standardized myocardial segmentation and nomenclature for tomographic imaging of the heart: a statement for healthcare professionals from the Cardiac Imaging Committee of the Council on Clinical Cardiology of the American Heart Association." *Circulation* 2002;105:539–42.

18. Hsia J, Klouj A, Prasad A, Burt J, Adams-Campbell L, Howard BV. "Progression of Coronary Calcification in Healthy Postmenopausal Women." *BMC Cardiovascular Disorders* 2004;4:21.

Heart Imaging

1. Tucker, K.J.; Cohen, T.J.; Botvinick, E.H.; Schiller, N.B. "The Applications of Adenosine in Non-Invasive Cardiac Imaging." *Herz* 1992; 17:122-136.

2. Foster, O'Kelly, B.; Tucker, K.J., et al. "Segmental Myocardial Viability can be Inferred from Combined Analysis of Echocardiographic Function and Scintigraphic Perfusion: Implications for 23-hour Perfusion and Positron Emission Tomographic Imaging." *J Am Coll Cardio* 1994.

3. "2006 Appropriateness Criteria for Cardiac Computed Tomography and Cardiac Magnetic Resonance Imaging." *JACC* Vol. 48, No. 7, 2006.

Risk Factors

1. Solfrizzi V, Capurso C, Colacicco AM, D'Introno A, Fontana C, Capurso SA, Torres F, Gadaleta AM, Koverech A, Capurso A, Panza F. "Efficacy and tolerability of combined treatment with l-carnitine and simvastatin in lowering lipoprotein(a) serum levels in patients with type 2 diabetes mellitus." *Atherosclerosis.* 2005 Dec 26; [Epub ahead of print]

2. Dreon DM, Fernstrom HA, Williams PT, Krauss RM. "A very low fat diet is not associated with improved lipoprotein profiles in men with a predominace of large LDLs." *Circulation* 1996;94:I-96.

3. Lamarche B, Tchernof A, Mauriege P, Cantin B, Dagenais R, Lupien PJ, Despres JP. Fasting insulin and apolipoprotein B levels and low-density lipoprotein particle size as risk factors for ischemic heart disease." *JAMA* 1998; 279:1955-1961.

4. Lamarche B, Tchernof A, Mauriege P, Cantin B, Dagenais GR, Lupien PJ, Despres JP. "Fasting insulin and apolipoprotein

B levels and low-density lipoprotein particle size as risk factor for ischemic heart disease." *JAMA* 1998;279:1955-1961.)

5. Desmarais, Rene L; Sarembock, Ian J, et al. "Elevated Serum Lipoprotein(a) Is a Risk Factor for Clinical Recurrence after Balloon Angioplasty." *Circulation.* 1995;91:1403-1409.

6. Mack WJ, Krauss RM, Hodis HN. "Lipoprotein subclasses in the Monitored Atherosclerosis Regression Study (MARS)." *Arterioscler Thromb Vasc Biol* 16 1996;16:697-704.

7. Hopkins P, Ellison R, Province M, Pankow J, Carr J, Arnett D, Lewis C, Heiss G, Hunt S. "Association of Coronary Calcified Plaque With Clinical Coronary Heart Disease in the National Heart, Lung and Blood Institute "Family Heart Study." *JACC* 2006, 99: 1564-1569.

Arrhythmias, Pacemakers and Defibrillators

1. "ACC/AHA/ESC 2006 Guidelines for Management of Patients With Ventricular Arrhythmias and the Prevention of Sudden Cardiac Death." *JACC*, Vol. 48, No. 5, 2006.

2. Cohen, T.J.; Tucker, K.J.; Abbot, J.A.; Botvinick, E.H.; Foster, E.; Schiller, N.B.; O'Connell, J.W.; Scheinman, M.M. "Usefulness of Adenosine in Augmenting Ventricular Pre-Excitation for Non-Invasive Localization of Accessory Pathways." *Am J Cardio* 1992; 1178-1185.

3. Cohen, T.J.; Tucker, K.J.; Lurie, K.G., et al. "Active Compression-Decompression (ACD): A New Method of Cardiopulmonary Resuscitation." *JAMA* 1992; 267:2916-2923.

4. Cohen, T.J.; Tucker, K.J.; Scheinman, M.M. "Accessory Pathway Identification via Adenosine Augmented Twelve-Lead Electrocardiogram." *J Arrhythmia Management* 1991; Summer: 3-8.

5. Cohen, T.J.; Tucker, K.J.; Redberg, R.F., et al. "Active Compression-Decompression Resuscitation: A Novel Method of Cardiopulmonary Resuscitation." *Am Heart J* 1992; 124:1145-1150.

6. Tucker, K.J.; Wilson, C. "A Comparison of Transesophageal Atrial Pacing and Direct Current Cardioversion for the Termination of Atrial Flutter: A Prospective, Randomized Clinical Trial." *Br Heart J* 1993; 69:530-535.

7. Tucker, K.J.; Redberg, R.F.; Ploss, D., et al. "Non-Invasive Assessment of the Pulmonary Artery Pressure Response to Exercise after Uncomplicated Heart Transplantation." *J Heart Lung Transplant* 1993; 12:604-612.

8. Tucker, K.J.; Redberg, R.F.; Schiller, N.; Cohen, T.J. "Active Compression-Decompression Resuscitation: Analysis of Transmitral Flow and Left Ventricular Volume by Transesophageal Echocardiography in Humans." *J Am Coll Cardio* 1993; 22:1485-93.

9. Tucker, K.J.; Cohen, T.J.; Scheinman, M.M. "Adenosine: Electrophysiologic Properties and Clinical Applications in Arrhythmia Management." *J Arrhythmia Management* 1993; Winter: 12-16.

10. Tucker, K.J.; Khan, J.H.; Savitt, M.A. "Active Compression-Decompression Resuscitation: Effects on Pulmonary Ventilation." *Resuscitation* 1993: 26:125-31.

11. Redberg, R.F.; Tucker, K.J.; Schiller, N.B. "The Role of Echocardiography During Cardiac Arrest." *Cardiol Clinics* 1993; 11:530-536.

12. Tucker, K.J.; Savitt, M.A.; Berrios, D.; Redberg, R.F. "Cardiopulmonary Resuscitation: Historical Perspectives, Physiology and New Direction." *Arch Intern Med* 1994; 154:2141-2150.

13. Tucker, K.J.; Galli, F.; Savitt, M.A.; Kahsai, D.; Bresnaham, L.; Redberg, R.F. "Active Compression-Decompression Resuscitation: Effects on Initial Return of Circulation and Survival after In-Hospital Cardiac Arrest." *J Am Coll Cardio* 1994; 24:201-9.

14. Tucker, K.J.; Kahn, J.; Idris, A.H.; Savitt, M.A. "The Bi-Phasic Mechanism of Cardiopulmonary Resuscitation: A physiologic Comparison of Active Compression-Decompression and High Impulse External Cardiac Massage." *Ann Emerg Med* 1994; 24:895-906.

15. Tucker, K.J.; Shaburihvili, T.S.; Gedevanishvili, A.T. "Manual External (Fist) Pacing during High Degree Atrioventricular Block: A Life-Saving Intervention." *Am J Emerg Med* 1994; 13:53-4.

16. Idris, A.H.; Tucker, K.J.; Fuerst, R.S.; Wenzel, V.; Banner, M.J. "Pulmonary Ventilation During Standard and Active Compression-Decompression Resuscitation." *Chest* 1995; in press.

17. Tucker, K.J.; Curtis, A.B.; Murphy, J.; Geiser, E.; Conti, C.R. "Transesophageal Echocardiographic Guidance during Transseptal Puncture for Radiofrequency Catheter Ablation of Left-Sided Accessory Pathways." *PACE* 1995; in press.

18. Haught, W.J.; Conti, J.B.; Tucker, K.J.; Curtis, A.B. "Emergency Intracardiac Defibrillation for Refractory Ventricular Fibrillation." *Clin Cardio* 1995; 18-109-11.

19. Tucker, K.J.; Curtis, A.B. "Advantages of Transesophageal Termination of Atrial Flutter with a Swallowable Pill Electrode." *Card Board Review* 1994; 11:43-47.

20. Tucker, K.J.; Larson, J.L.; Curtis, A.B. "Advanced Cardiac Life Support: Update on Recent Guidelines and a Look into the Future." *Clin Cardio* 1995; 18:497-504.

21. Wenzel, V.; Idris, A.H.; Fuerst, R.S.; Banner, M.J.; Tucker, K.J. "The Composition of Gas Given by Mouth-to-Mouth Ventilation during Cardiopulmonary Resuscitation." *Chest* 1994; 106:1806-10.

22. Conti, J.B.; Tucker, K.J.; Mines, M.H.; Curtis, A.B. "Radiofrequency Ablation of the Sinus Node for Inappropriate Sinus Tachycardia." Submitted for publication.

23. Tucker, K.J.; Santora, L.J.; Smith, D.H.M.; Cobb, T.C. "Advances in Cardiopulmonary Resuscitation." *Primary Cardiology* 1995; in press.

24. Tucker, K.J.; Santora, L.J.; Smith, D.H.M.; Cobb, T.C. "Physical Limitations during Performance of Cardiopulmonary Resuscitation: A Comparison of Standard, High Impulse and Active Compression-Decompression Methods." *Resuscitation* 1995; in press.

25. Cohen, T.J.; Noubani, H.; Tucker, K.J.; Quan, W.; Trazzera, S.; Stern, G. "Active Compression-Decompression Defibrillation (ACD2) Provides Effective Defibrillation during Cardiopulmonary Resuscitation." Submitted for publication.

26. Tucker, K.J.; Cannom, D.S.; Lerman, L.; Bhandari, A.K. "Cardiac Rhythm Disorders and Antiarrhythmic Drug Therapy during Pregnancy." Submitted for publication.

27. Curtis, A.B.; Conti, J.B.; Reilly, R.E.; Tucker, K.J. "Implantable Cardioverter-Defibrillators (ICDs): Should Patients be Allowed to Drive?" *J Am Coll Cardio* 1995; 26:180-4.

28. Tucker, K.J.; Law, J.; Rodrigues, M. "Treatment of Refractory Recurrent Multifocal Atrial Tachycardia with Atrioventricular Junction Ablation and Permanent Pacing." *J Invas Cardio* 1995; 7:207-12.

Congestive Heart Failure

1. Koelling TM, Chen RS, Lubwama RN, L'Italien GJ, Eagle KA. "The expanding national burden of heart failure in the United States: the influence of heart failure in women." *Am Heart J.* 2004; 147: 74–78.

2. Hunt SA, Baker DW, Chin MH, et al. "ACC/AHA guidelines for the evaluation and management of chronic heart failure in the adult: executive summary: a report of the American College of Cardiology/American Heart Association Task Force on Practice Guidelines" (Committee to revise the 1995 Guidelines for the Evaluation and Management of Heart Failure). *J Am Coll Cardiol.* 2001; 38: 2101–2113.

3. Baik HK, Budoff MJ, Lane KL, Bakhsheshi H, Brundage BH. "Accurate measures of left ventricular ejection fraction using electron beam tomography: a comparison with radionuclide angiography, and cine angiography." *Int J Card Imaging* 2000;16:391–8.

4. Vijayaraghavan K, Santora L, Kahn J, et al. "New graduated pressure regimen for external counterpulsation reduces mortality and improves outcomes in congestive heart failure: a report from the cardiomedics external counterpulsation patient registry." *Congest Heart Fail.* 2005;11:147-152.

Hormone Replacement Related

1. Barnabei VM, Cochrane BB, Aragaki AK, Nygaard I, Williams RS, McGovern PG, Young RL, Wells EC, O'Sullivan MJ, Chen B, Schenken R, Johnson SR. "Menopausal Symptoms and Treatment-Related Effects of Estrogen and Progestin in the Women's Health Initiative." *Obstet Gynecol* 2005;105:1063-73.

2. Bonds D, Lasser N, Qi L, Brzyski R, Caan B, Heiss G, Limacher MC, Liu JG, Mason E, Oberman A, O'Sullivan MJ, Phillips LS,

Prineas RJ, Tinker L. "The Effect of Conjugated Equine Oestrogen on Diabetes Incidence: The Women's Health Initiative Randomised Trial." *Diabetologia* 2006;49:459-468.

3. Brunner RL, Gass M, Aragaki A, Hays J, Granek I, Woods N, Mason E, Brzyski R, Ockene J, Assaf A, LaCroix A, Matthews K, Wallace R. "Effects of Conjugated Equine Estrogen on Health-Related Quality of Life in Postmenopausal Women with Hysterectomy: Results from the Women's Health Initiative Randomized Clinical Trial." *Arch Intern Med* 2005;165:1976-1986.

4. Cauley JA, Robbins J, Chen Z, Cummings SR, Jackson RD, LaCroix AZ, LeBoff M, Lewis CE, McGowan J, Neuner J, Pettinger M, Stefanick ML, Wactawski-Wende J, Watts NB. "Effects of Estrogen Plus Progestin on Risk of Fracture and Bone Mineral Density." *JAMA* 2003;290(13):1729-1738.

5. Chen Z, Bassford T, Green SB, Cauley JA, Jackson RD, LaCroix AZ, Leboff M, Stefanick ML, Margolis KL. "Postmenopausal Hormone Therapy and Body Composition—A Substudy of the Estrogen Plus Progestin Trial of the Women's Health Initiative." *Am J Clin Nutr* 2005;82:651-6.

6. Chlebowski R, Hendrix SL, Langer RD, Stefanick M, Gass M, Lane D, Rodabough R, Gilligan MA, Cyr M, Thomson C, Khandekar J, Petrovitch H, McTiernan A. "Influence of Estrogen Plus Progestin on Breast Cancer and Mammography in Healthy Postmenopausal Women: the Women's Health Initiative Randomized Trial." *JAMA* 2003;289:3243-3253.

7. Hsia J, Langer RD, Manson JE, Kuller L, Johnson KC, Hendrix SL, Pettinger M, Heckbert SR, Greep N, Crawford S, Eaton CB, Kostis JB, Caralis P, Prentice R. "Conjugated Equine Estrogens and Coronary Heart Disease: The Women's Health Initiative." *Arch Intern Med* 2006;166:357-365.

8. Barrett-Connor E, Grady D. "Hormone replacement therapy,

heart disease, and other considerations." *Annu Rev Public Health.* 1998;19:55–72.

9. Anderson GL, Judd HL, Kaunitz AM, Barad DH, Beresford SAA, Pettinger M, Jiu J, McNeeley SG, Lopez AM. "Effects of Estrogen Plus Progestin on Gynecologic Cancers and Associated Diagnostic Procedures: The Women's Health Initiative Randomized Trial." *JAMA* 2003;290:1739-1748.

External Counterpulsation

1. Vijayaraghavan K, Santora L, Kahn J, et al. "New graduated pressure regimen for external counterpulsation reduces mortality and improves outcomes in congestive heart failure: a report from the cardiomedics external counterpulsation patient registry." *Congest Heart Fail.* 2005;11:147-152.

2. Lawson WE, Kennard ED, Hui JC, Holubkov R, Kelsey SF. "Analysis of baseline factors associated with reduction in chest pain in patients with angina pectoris treated by enhanced external counterpulsation." *Am J Cardiol.* 2003;92:439–443. doi: 10.1016/S0002-9149(03)00662-3.

3. Lawson WE, Hui JC, Kennard ED, Barsness G, Kelsey SF. "Predictors of benefit in angina patients one year after completing enhanced external counterpulsation: initial responders to treatment versus nonresponders." *Cardiology.* 2005;103:201–206. doi: 10.1159/000085170.

4. Niebauer J, Cooke JP. "Cardiovascular effects of exercise: role of endothelial shear stress." *J Am Coll Cardiol.* 1996;28:1652–1660. doi: 10.1016/S0735-1097(96)00393-2.

5. Bonetti PO, Barsness GW, Keelan PC, Schnell TI, Pumper GM, Kuvin JT, Schnall RP, Holmes DR, Higano ST, Lerman A. "Enhanced external counterpulsation improves endothelial function in patients with symptomatic coronary artery disease." *J Am*

Coll Cardiol. 2003;41:1761–1768. doi: 10.1016/S0735-1097(03)00329-2.

6. Arora RR, Chou TM, Jain D, Fleishman B, Crawford L, McKiernan T, Nesto R, Ferrans CE, Keller S. "Effects of enhanced external counterpulsation on Health-Related Quality of Life continue 12 months after treatment: a substudy of the Multicenter Study of Enhanced External Counterpulsation." *J Investig Med.* 2002;50:25–32.

Heart Attack Related

1. Norris CM, Ghali WA, Galbraith PD, Graham MM, Jensen LA, Knudtson ML. "Women with coronary artery disease report worse health-related quality of life outcomes compared to men." *Health Qual Life Outcomes.* 2004; 2: 21. published online. May 5, 2004, PMCID: 420257.

2. Koek HL, de Bruin A, Gast F, Gevers E, Kardaun JWPF, Reitsma JB, Grobbee DE, Bots ML. "Short- and Long-Term Prognosis After Acute Myocardial Infarction in Men Versus Women." *Am J Cardiol* , pages 993-999,18 August 2006.

3. Jiang SL, Ji XP, Zhao YX, Wang XR, Song ZF, Ge ZM, Guo T, Zhang C, Zhang Y. "Predictors of In-Hospital Mortality Difference Between Male and Female Patients With Acute Myocardial Infarction." *Am J Cardiol.* pages 1000-1003, 21 August 2006.

4. Hsia J, Aragaki A, Bloch M, LaCroix AZ, Wallace R. "Predictors of Angina Pectoris Versus Myocardial Infarction from the Women's Health Initiative Observational Study." *Am J Cardiol* 2004; 93:673-678.

5. American Heart Association. Heart Disease and Stroke Statistics: 2005 Update. Dallas, Tex: American Heart Association; 2005.

Heart Valve Related

1. Tucker, K.J.; Johnson, J.; Ong, T., et al. "Medical Management of Prosthetic Aortic Valve Endocarditis and Aortic Root Abscess." *Am Heart J* 1993; 125:1195-7.

2. Shavelle DM, Takasu J, Budoff MJ, Mao S, Zhao XQ, O'Brien KD. "HMG CoA reductase inhibitor (statin) and aortic valve calcium." *Lancet* 2002;359:1125–6.

3. ACC/AHA 2006 Guidelines for the Management of Patients With Valvular Heart Disease JACC, Vol. 48, No. 3, 2006.

Diet Related

1. Santora LJ, Butkus D, Armentrout S, *The OC Cure For Heart Disease.* OC Heart Health Books, Orange County, California, 2006.

2. Gazzaniga, DA, Fowler, M, Moloo, J. *The No Salt Lowest Sodium Cookbook series*, St. Martin's Press, www.megaheart.com.

3. "Clinical guidelines on the identification, evaluation, and treatment of overweight and obesity in adults — the Evidence Report." *Obes Res* 1998;6:Suppl 2:51S-209S. [Erratum, Obes Res 1998;6:464.]

4. Thomas PR, ed. *Weighing the options: criteria for evaluating weight-management programs*. Washington, DC: National Academy Press, 1995.

5. "Position of the American Dietetic Association: weight management." *J Am Diet Assoc* 1997;97:71-74.

6. Krauss RM, Deckelbaum RJ, Ernst N, et al. "Dietary guidelines for healthy American adults: a statement for health professionals from the National Committee, American Heart Association." *Circulation* 1996;94:1795-1800.

7. Steward HL, Bethea MC, Andrews SS, Balart LA. *Sugar busters!* New York: Ballantine Books, 1995.

8. Eades MR, Eades MD. *Protein power.* New York: Bantam Books, 1999.

9. Atkins RC. *Dr. Atkins' new diet revolution.* Rev. ed. New York: Avon Books, 1998.

10. Sears B, Lawren B. *The Zone: a dietary road map to lose weight permanently, reset your genetic code, prevent disease, achieve maximum physical performance.* New York: HarperCollins, 1995.

11. Heller RF, Heller RF. *The carbohydrate addict's diet: the lifelong solution to yo-yo dieting.* New York: New American Library, 1993.

12. Stein K. "High-protein, low-carbohydrate diets: do they work?" *J Am Diet Assoc* 2000;100:760-761.

13. St Jeor ST, Howard BV, Prewitt TE, Bovee V, Bazzarre T, Eckel RH. "Dietary protein and weight reduction: a statement for healthcare professionals from the nutrition committee of the Council on Nutrition, Physical Activity, and Metabolism of the American Heart Association." *Circulation* 2001;104:1869-1874.

14. American Heart Association statement on high-protein, low-carbohydrate diet study presented at scientific sessions, November 19, 2002. Chicago: American Heart Association, 2002.

15. High-protein diets: AHA recommendation. Chicago: American Heart Association, 2006.

16. Willett WC, Sampson L, Stampfer MJ, et al. "Reproducibility and validity of a semiquantitative food frequency questionnaire." *Am J Epidemiol* 1985;122:51-65.

17. Willett WC. *Nutritional epidemiology.* 2nd ed. New York: Oxford University Press, 1998.

18. Composition of foods: raw, processed, prepared. Washington, DC: Department of Agriculture, 1993.

19. Liu S, Willett WC, Stampfer MJ, et al. "A prospective study of dietary glycemic load, carbohydrate intake, and risk of coronary heart disease in US women." *Am J Clin Nutr* 2000;71:1455-1461.

20. Rimm EB, Stampfer MJ, Colditz GA, Chute CG, Litin LB, Willett WC. "Validity of self reported waist and hip circumferences in men and women." *Epidemiology* 1990;1:466-473.

21. Hu FB, Manson JE, Stampfer MJ, et al. "Diet, lifestyle, and the risk of type 2 diabetes mellitus in women." *N Engl J Med* 2001;345:790-797.

22. Rose GA, Blackburn H. Cardiovascular survey methods. WHO monograph series no. 58. Geneva: World Health Organization, 1982.

23. Stampfer MJ, Willett WC, Speizer FE, et al. "Test of the National Death Index." *Am J Epidemiol* 1984;119:837-839.

24. Hu FB, Stampfer MJ, Manson JA, et al. "Dietary fat intake and the risk of coronary heart disease in women." *N Engl J Med* 1997;337:1491-1499.

25. Cox DR, Oakes D. Analysis of survival data. London: Chapman & Hall, 1984.

26. Halton TL, Hu FB. "The effects of high protein diets on thermogenesis, satiety and weight loss: a critical review." *J Am Coll Nutr* 2004;23:373-385.

27. Nordmann AJ, Nordmann A, Briel M, et al. "Effects of low-carbohydrate vs low-fat diets on weight loss and cardiovascular risk factors: a meta-analysis of randomized controlled trials." *Arch Intern Med* 2006;166:285-293. [Erratum, *Arch Intern Med* 2006;166:932.]

28. McGee DL, Reed DM, Yano K, Kagan A, Tillotson J. "Ten-year incidence of coronary heart disease in the Honolulu Heart Program: relationship to nutrient intake." *Am J Epidemiol* 1984;119:667-676.

29. Kushi LH, Lew RA, Stare FJ, et al. "Diet and 20-year mortality from coronary heart disease: the Ireland-Boston Diet-Heart Study." *N Engl J Med* 1985;312:811-818.

30. Ascherio A, Rimm EB, Giovannucci EL, Spiegelman D, Stampfer MJ, Willett WC. "Dietary fat and risk of coronary heart disease in men: cohort follow up study in the United States." *BMJ* 1996;313:84-90.

31. Pietinen P, Ascherio A, Korhonen P, et al. "Intake of fatty acids and risk of coronary heart disease in a cohort of Finnish men: the Alpha-Tocopherol, Beta-Carotene Cancer Prevention Study." *Am J Epidemiol* 1997;145:876-887.

32. Oomen CM, Ocke MC, Feskens JM, van Erp-Baarrt MJ, Kok FJ, Kromhout D. "Association between trans fatty acid intake and 10-year risk of coronary heart disease in the Zutphen Elderly Study: a prospective population-based study." *Lancet* 2001;357:746-751.

33. Howard BV, Van Horn L, Hsia J, et al. "Low-fat dietary pattern and risk of cardiovascular disease: the Women's Health Initiative Randomized Controlled Dietary Modification Trial." *JAMA* 2006;295:655-666.

34. Hu FB, Willett WC. "Optimal diets for prevention of coronary heart disease." *JAMA* 2002;288:2569-2578.

35. Hu FB, Stampfer MJ, Manson JE, et al. "Dietary protein and risk of ischemic heart disease in women." *Am J Clin Nutr* 1999;70:221-227.

36. Ludwig DS. "The glycemic index: physiological mechanisms relating to obesity, diabetes, and cardiovascular disease." *JAMA* 2002;287:2414-2423.

37. Knight EL, Stampfer MJ, Hankinson SE, Spiegelman D, Curhan GC. "The impact of protein intake on renal function decline in women with normal renal function or mild renal insufficiency." *Ann Intern Med* 2003;138:460-467.

Addendum B
Useful Web Sites

Orange County Heart Institute and Research Center : www.ocheart.org Description: The site for the authors' Heart Institute. Description of their clinical practice, latest research, and treatments available at the Institute.

Orange County Vital Imaging : www.ocvitalimaging.com Description: The site for the authors' imaging center. OC Vital Imaging provides cardiac CT imaging. A description of the technology and various services is described.

OC Cure For Heart Disease: www.ocheartcure.com Description: The site for the authors' other book, *The OC Cure for Heart Disease.* Co-authored by Dick Butkus (NFL Hall of Fame), and Steve Armentrout MD, describes an approach to heart disease using EBCT scan technology.

Megaheart Low Sodium Dietary Plan For Heart Disease: www.megaheart.com. Support for No Salt, Lowest Sodium Cookbook series for heart disease and other chronic illnesses requiring a low sodium lifestyle.

Ask NOAH About: Women's Health: www.noah-health.org/ english/wellness/healthyliving/womenshealth.html Description: The New York Online Access to Health (NOAH) is a bilingual (English and Spanish) health information site.

HHS U.S. Food and Drug Administration (FDA) Office of Women's Health (OWH): www.fda.gov/womens/ Description: The mission of the FDA's Office of Women's Health (OWH) is "to serve as a champion for women's health both within and outside the agency."

Health Resources and Services Administration (HRSA): Women's Health: www.hrsa.gov/womenshealth/default.htm Details: The Health Resources and Services Administration (HRSA), an agency of the U.S. Department of Health & Human Services (HHS), provides links to women's health contacts.

HHS Office on Women's Health: 4woman.gov/owh/index.htm Description: "The Office on Women's Health (OWH) in the Department of Health & Human Services (HHS) is the government's champion and focal point for women's health issues."

HHS Office of Women's Health (OWH): National Women's Health Information Center : 4woman.gov Description: The National Women's Health Information Center, a service of the Office on Women's Health in the Department of Health & Human Services. Disabilities, body image, men's health, minority health information, and other topics.

National Women's Health Resource Center (NWHRC): www.healthywomen.org/ Description: The National Women's Health Resource Center (NWHRC) is a non-profit, national clearinghouse for women's health information.

NIH Office of Research on Women's Health: www4.od.nih.gov/orwh/ Description: Links are given to reports (e.g.: Agenda for Research on Women's Health for the 21st Century: Executive Summary).

Society for Women's Health Research: www.womens-health.org/ Description: Nonprofit advocacy group "promotes the inclusion of women in medical research studies and encourages the scientific examination of the basic biological and physiological differences between men and women, and how those differences affect both health and disease."

WebMD Healthy Women: my.webmd.com/living_better/her Description: WebMD is an online information, research, educational services and communities for consumers and physicians.

The North American Menopause Society: www.menopause.org/ Description: A scientific nonprofit organization devoted to promoting women's health during midlife and beyond through an understanding of menopause. Information is provided for health care consumers and professionals alike.

Glossary

Ablation also called RFA
Radio Frequency Ablation - catheter is in place inside the heart, tiny areas of the heart are "burned" by radio-frequency energy to cure arrhythmia.

ACE (angiotensin-converting enzyme) inhibitor
A medication that opens up blood vessels, making it easier for the heart to pump, used for congestive heart failure and to lower blood pressure.

Acute Coronary Syndrome
General name for all patients who have serious chest pain, whether it is from a heart attack or from unstable angina.

Anastomosis
A surgical connection, often between two blood vessels.

Aneurysm
A thin, weakened area in a blood vessel or area of the heart.

Angiography
An x-ray study that uses dye injected into arteries to study blood circulation.

Angina
Chest pain often caused by lack blood flow to the heart - there are several different categories of angina.

Angioedema
Swelling involving the skin and its layers, the mucous membranes and sometimes even internal organs. ACE inhibitors can cause angioedema, particularly of the throat and mouth.

Angiogenesis
Growth of new blood vessels to bring blood to tissue

Angiogram
X-rays of the heart's arteries, using a catheter procedure and dye, or CT scan and dye.

Angioplasty
A non-surgical procedure for treating narrowed arteries.

Angiotensin II
A protein that is a vasoconstrictor. It is formed from angiotensin 1 by the action of ACE inside the lungs. Angiotensin II is over-active in heart failure and has harmful effects on the heart. ACE inhibitors and ARBs reduce these effects.

Anticoagulant
A medication that keeps blood from clotting.

Antihypertensive
A medication that lowers blood pressure.

Antioxidant
A substance that reduces damage from free radicals.

Annuloplasty
Surgery in which a synthetic ring is placed around the rim of a heart valve (annulus). This causes proper closing by shrinking the size of the valve opening.

Aorta
The largest artery in the body and the primary blood vessel which carries oxygenated blood out of the heart to the rest of the body.

Aortic arch
The curved portion of the aorta (the large blood vessel that carries oxygen-rich blood away from the heart to the body).

Aortic regurgitation or insufficiency
Backwards leakage of blood from the aorta, through a weakened aortic valve, and into the left ventricle, resulting in stress in the left heart and inadequate blood flow to the body.

Aortic stenosis
Narrowing of the opening of the aortic valve (the valve that regulates blood flow from the left ventricle into the aorta).

Aortic valve
The valve that regulates blood flow from the heart into the aorta.

ARB
Angiotensin II Receptor Blocker. Also called angiotensin antagonists. ARBs reduce angiotensin II but do it at the cell wall instead of in the blood stream inside the lungs like ACE inhibitors.

Arginine
An amino acid that promotes nitric oxide in the artery lining, which then causes arteries to dilate.

Arrhythmia (Also called dysrhythmia)
A fast, slow, or irregular heartbeat.

Arterioles
Small branches of arteries.

Artery
A blood vessel that carries oxygenated blood away from the heart to the body.

Arteriosclerosis
Commonly called "hardening of the arteries"; a variety of conditions caused by fatty or calcium deposits in the artery walls causing them to thicken.

Atrial fibrillation
A very fast and irregular beating of the atria (the upper two chambers of the heart).

Atrial flutter
A very fast beating of the atria (the upper two chambers of the heart).

Atrial septal defect (ASD)
A hole in the wall between the right and left atria (the two upper chambers of the heart).

Atrial septum
The wall between the right and left atria (the two upper chambers of the heart).

Atrium One of two upper chambers in the heart.

Atrioventricular block
An interruption of the electrical signal between the atria and the ventricles.

Atrioventricular (AV) node
A cluster of cells between the atria and ventricles that regulate the electrical current.

Bacterial endocarditis
A bacterial infection of the valves and interior surfaces of the heart.

Balloon angioplasty (PTCA)
A procedure usually done in the cardiac catheterization laboratory that uses a catheter (tube) with a balloon in the tip to open up a narrowed valve or blood vessel.

Beating heart bypass surgery
An operation that repairs problems involving the blood vessels attached to the heart, and may not need the use of the heart-lung bypass machine.

Beta blocker
A medication that limits the activity of epinephrine (a hormone that increases blood pressure).

Bicuspid
A valve that has two leaflets.

BiV (biventricular)
Controlling the heart's beating using a special pacemaker with 3 leads - one in the right atrium, one in right ventricle and one in a coronary vein of the left ventricle. Thus control of both ventricles.

Blood clot
A thick, gelled mass of blood, also called a thrombus.

Blood pressure
The force or pressure exerted by the heart when pumping blood; the pressure of blood in the arteries.

BNP (B-type Natriuretic Peptide)
A natural hormone the heart releases when it cannot pump sufficient blood and is an indication of congestive heart failure.

Bradycardia
Abnormally slow heartbeat.

Bundle-branch block
A condition in which the heart's electrical system is unable to normally conduct the electrical signal through one of the two electrical pathways that connect the top chambers (atrium) and the bottom chambers(ventricules).

CABG

Coronary Artery Bypass Grafting, often called bypass surgery. Blood vessels are taken from other parts of your body during surgery (usually thighs) and sewn into coronary arteries to replace "bad" sections, thus restoring proper blood flow to your heart.

CAD

Coronary Artery Disease - condition that reduces blood flow through the coronary arteries to the heart muscle. Usually caused by plaque buildup in the arteries ("blocked" arteries.)

Calcium channel blocker

A medication that lowers blood pressure and relaxes the artery walls.

Capillaries

Tiny blood vessels between arteries and veins that distribute oxygen-rich blood to the body.

Cardiac

Pertaining to the heart.

Cardiac arrest

The stopping of heartbeat.

Cardiac catheterization

A diagnostic procedure in which a tiny, hollow tube (catheter) is inserted into an artery or vein in order to evaluate the heart and blood vessels.

Cardiac output

The amount of blood that goes through the circulatory system in one minute.

Cardiologist

A physician who specializes in the medical evaluation and treatment of heart diseases.

Cardiology

The clinical study and practice of treating the heart.

Cardiomegaly

Enlargement of the heart.

Cardiomyopathy

A disease of the heart muscle that causes it to lose its pumping strength. The heart walls can be excessively thickened or excessively thin.

Cardiovascular (CV)
Pertaining to the heart and blood vessel (circulatory) system.

Cardioversion
The procedure of applying electrical shock to the chest to change an abnormal heartbeat into a normal one.

Cardiac troponin I
An enzyme released from the heart muscle if there is heart muscle damage from a heart attack or congestive heart failure or inflammation of the heart and other factors.

Carotid artery
The major arteries in the neck that supply blood to the brain.

Catheter
A small, thin tube; may refer to a tube used during a cardiac catheterization procedure to inject dye, obtain blood samples, and measure pressures inside the heart; may also refer to a small tube used to help drain the bladder during and after a surgical procedure.

CCB
Calcium Channel Blocker. These drugs have numerous functions: control high blood pressure, control certain types of abnormal heart rhythms, and control angina. Includes amlodipine (Norvasc, Lotrel), diltiazem (Cardizem), and verapamil (Covera, Isoptin, Calan).

Cholesterol
A waxy substance that is produced by the human body. It is also found in animal fats, shellfish, and in dairy products (such as beef, chicken, pork, butter, milk, cheese, and eggs). It is not found in plant products.

Cineangiography
The procedure of taking moving pictures to show the passage of dye through blood vessels during invasive coronary angiograms.

Circulatory system
Pertaining to the heart and blood vessels and the circulation of blood.

Claudication
Unusual pain in the calf or back of thigh or buttocks area during walking, often caused by blockage of blood vessels in the legs.

Coarctation of the aorta
A congenital heart defect that results in narrowing of the aorta.

Collateral vessels
New blood vessels that are created by the body to provide extra blood flow to an area when the blood vessel(s) that are already there are too small, narrowed, or blocked.

Computerized tomography scan (also called CT or CAT scan)
A non-invasive xray that takes cross-sectional images of the body and heart or other internal organs; a computer reconstructs the xray to form a three dimensional image. EBCT and MDCT are the two common types of CT scans.

Conduction system
The electrical system inside the heart that stimulates the heart to beat.

Congenital
Present at birth.

Congenital heart defect
A heart problem present at birth, caused by improper development of the heart during fetal development.

Congestive heart failure
A condition in which the heart cannot pump out all of the blood that enters it; this leads to an accumulation of blood in the vessels leading to the heart and fluid in the body tissues. Excess blood in the pulmonary (lung) blood vessels occurs, leading to "congestion" in the lungs.

COPD
Chronic obstructive pulmonary disease, a long term scarring of the lungs usually due to tobacco abuse.

Coronary arteries
Two arteries that come from the aorta to provide blood to the heart muscle.

COX inhibitor
Cyclooxygenase - an enzyme inhibited by NSAIDs. COX-1 protects the lining of the stomach. COX-2 causes pain and inflammation. Newer NSAIDs like Celebrex only block COX-2 while older NSAIDs like ibuprofen block both.

Cyanosis
Insufficient oxygen in the blood, causing blue discoloration of skin and lips.

Defibrillator
An electronic device used to establish normal heartbeat.

Dilate
Enlarge. A dilated heart is an enlarged heart.

Distal
Farthest-as in, the distal artery is the artery farthest away from the catheter.

Diastole
The time during each heartbeat when the ventricles are at rest, filling with blood and not pumping.

Diastolic blood pressure
The lowest blood pressure measure in the arteries, which occurs between heartbeats.

Diuretic
A medication that helps the kidneys to remove excess fluids from the body, lowering blood pressure as well as decreasing edema (swelling).

Diuresis
Increased urination.

Doppler ultrasound
A procedure that uses sound waves to evaluate heart, blood vessels, and valves.

Dyspnea
Shortness of breath.

Dysrhythmia
An abnormal heart rhythm.

ECP
External counterpulsation. A non-invasive method to improve blood flow to the heart to reduce angina. Inflatable cuffs on the legs improve blood flow to the heart.

Echocardiogram (echo)
A procedure that evaluates the structure and function of the heart by using sound waves recorded on an electronic sensor which produce a moving picture of the heart and heart valves.

Edema
Swelling; abnormal accumulation of fluid in body tissues, usually causing swelling in the legs.

Effusion
A collection of fluid in a closed cavity, usually in the lining around the lungs or around the heart.

Ejection Fraction
Percentage of blood in the left ventricle that is pumped out in one beat.

Electrocardiogram (ECG or EKG)
A test that records the electrical activity of the heart, shows abnormal rhythms (arrhythmias or dysrhythmias), and detects heart muscle stress.

Electrophysiological study (EPS)
A cardiac catheterization to study electrical current in patients who have arrhythmias.

Endocardium
The membrane that covers the inside surface of the heart.

Endocarditis
A bacterial infection of the valves and interior surfaces of the heart.

End-to-end anastomosis
Surgical connection of two segments of blood vessel by stitching the open end of one segment to the open end of another segment.

Enlarged heart
A condition of the heart in which it is larger than normal.

Epicardium
The membrane that covers the outside of the heart.

Exercise electrocardiogram (ECG or EKG)
A test to assess the cardiac rhythm and function by having the person exercise on a treadmill or bicycle.

Fibrillation
Rapid contractions of the heart muscles.

Fibrosis
A condition of increased connective tissue containing or made up of tissue resembling fibers.

Free radical
Oxygen atom with an odd number of electrons. It seeks other molecules to steal an electron from so it can balance its electron pairs. This thieving damages the molecules it steals from.

Fluoroscopy
An x-ray procedure that takes continuous pictures to evaluate moving structures within the body, such as the heart.

Flutter
Ineffective contractions of the heart muscles.

Foramen ovale
A hole between the right and left atria, present in all unborn children, that remains open after birth for variable periods of time.

Heart attack (also called myocardial infarction)
Occurs when one or more regions of the heart muscle experience a severe or prolonged decrease in oxygen supply caused by a blocked blood flow to the heart muscle.

Heart block
Interrupted electrical impulse to heart muscles.

Heart-lung bypass machine
A machine that performs for the heart and lungs during open heart surgery.

Heart valve prolapse
A condition of the heart valve in which it buckles backwards and does not fully close, causing regurgitation of blood from one heart chamber to the next.

Hematoma
A bruise. A "pool" of blood-usually clotted-in an organ, space, or tissue, due to a break in a blood vessel wall.

High blood pressure (also called hypertension)
Blood pressure that is above the normal range.

High density lipoprotein (HDL)
The "good" cholesterol that promotes breakdown and removal of cholesterol from the body.

Holter monitor
A portable EKG machine worn for a 24-hour period or longer to evaluate irregular, fast, or slow heart rhythms while engaging in normal activities.

Homograft
A blood vessel taken from a tissue donor, used to replace a defective blood vessel, most often the pulmonary artery or aorta.

Hypertrophic obstructive cardiomyopathy (also called HOCM, hypertrophic cardiomyopathy, asymmetrical septal hypertrophy, or ASH, or idiopathic hypertrophic subaortic stenosis or IHSS)
Enlarged and thickened heart muscle that causes impeded blood flow. The condition can cause breathlessness, chest pain and sudden death.

Hypotension
Low blood pressure.

Hypoxia
Abnormal oxygen content in the organs and tissues of the body.

Inferior vena cava
The large blood vessel (vein) that returns blood from the legs and abdomen to the heart.

Insufficiency
A valve deformity that allows the blood to leak backwards when the valve is closed.

Ischemia
Decreased flow of oxygenated blood to an organ due to obstruction in an artery.

Ischemic heart disease
Coronary artery disease or coronary heart disease caused by narrowing of the coronary arteries and decreased blood flow to the heart.

Jugular veins
Veins that carry blood from the head back to the heart. These are visible at the side of the neck next to the carotid arteries.

Kawasaki disease
An immune system disorder affecting the heart, particularly the coronary arteries.

Left atrium
The upper left-hand chamber of the heart. It receives oxygen-rich (red) blood from the lungs via the four pulmonary veins, and then sends this blood to the left ventricle.

LBBB
Left Bundle Branch Block, an electrical disorder of the heart.

Left ventricle
The lower left-hand chamber of the heart. It receives oxygen-rich (red) blood from the left atrium and pumps it into the aorta, which takes the blood to the body. The left ventricle must be strong and muscular in order to pump enough blood to the body to meet its requirements.

Lesion
An injury or wound.

Lipid
A fatty substance in the blood.

Lipoproteins
Transporters of fatty substances in the blood.

Low density lipoprotein (LDL)
The primary cholesterol-carrying substance in the body. In large amounts, it accumulates inside arteries.

Lumen
The hollow area inside a blood vessel.

Magnetic resonance imaging (MRI)
A diagnostic procedure that uses a combination of large magnets, radiofrequencies, and a computer to produce detailed images of organs and structures within the body.

Marfan syndrome
A genetic disorder which affects the connective tissue of the body. It causes dilation of blood vessels and abnormalities of cardiac valves and the thoracic aorta.

Mechanical valve
An artificial valve used to replace a diseased or defective valve, usually made of metal, most often the aortic valve and mitral valve.

Median sternotomy
An incision in the center of the chest, from the top to the bottom of the breastbone, used for many congenital heart defect repair surgeries.

Mitral valve
The valve that controls blood flow between the left atrium and left ventricle in the heart.

Mitral valve prolapse (MVP)
An abnormality of the valve between the left atrium and left ventricle of the heart that causes backward flow of blood from the left ventricle into the left atrium.

Monounsaturated fats
Dietary fats, such as olive oil or canola oil, that may lower LDL cholesterol levels.

MUGA
Multiple Gated Acquisition or radionuclide ventriculography. An x-ray of heart function using an injection of radioactives.

Murmur
A blowing or rasping sound heard while listening to the heart that may or may not indicate problems within the heart or circulatory system.

Myocardial infarction (Also called heart attack)
Occurs when one or more regions of the heart muscle experience a severe or prolonged decrease in oxygen supply caused by a blocked blood flow to the heart muscle.

Myocardial ischemia
Insufficient blood flow to part of the heart.

Myocarditis
Inflammation of the heart muscles.

Myocardium
The muscular layer of the heart.

Noninvasive procedure
A diagnostic effort or treatment that does not require entering the body or puncturing the skin.

NSAID
Non-Steroidal Anti-Inflammatory Drug – Ibuprofen and naproxen are examples.

Obesity
Overweight by 30 percent of the ideal body weight.

Occluded artery
An artery that is narrowed by plaque that impedes blood flow.

Open heart surgery
Surgery that involves opening the chest and heart while a heart-lung machine performs for the heart and lungs during the operation.

Orthostatic
From standing. Orthostatic hypotension is low blood pressure when you're standing.

Orthopnea
Inability to breathe except in an upright position. This is a symptom of congestive heart failure.

Oxygen desaturation
Insufficient amounts of oxygen in the bloodstream. Desaturation can occur when a person has congestive heart failure or numerous types of lung disease. Normal oxygen saturation in the arteries is 95 to 100 percent.

Oxygen saturation
The extent to which the hemoglobin is saturated with oxygen. (Hemoglobin is an element in the bloodstream that binds with oxygen and carries it to the organs and tissues of the body.) A normal oxygen saturation of the blood leaving the heart to the body is 95 to 100 percent. The oxygen saturation of the blood returning to the heart after delivering oxygen to the body is 75 percent.

Pacemaker
An electronic device that is surgically placed in the patient's body and connected to the heart to regulate the heartbeat.

Palpitation
A sensation in the chest caused by an irregular heartbeat.

Patent
Open.

Patent ductus arteriosus (PDA)
A blood vessel present in all infants that usually closes shortly after birth. It connects the aorta to the pulmonary artery. When it remains open, it allows extra blood to pass through from the aorta to the lungs.

Patent foramen ovale
An opening in the atrial septum (wall between the right and left atria) that is present in all infants, but which usually closes shortly after birth. When it remains open, it allows extra blood to pass through the opening from the left atrium to the right atrium.

Pericardial effusion
A build up of excess fluid in between the heart and the membrane that surrounds it, often due to inflammation.

Pericarditis
An inflammation or infection of the sac which surrounds the heart.

Pericardiocentesis
A diagnostic procedure that uses a needle to draw fluid from the pericardium.

Pericardium
The membrane that surrounds the heart.

Plaque
Deposits of fat or other substances attached to the artery wall.

Platelets
Cells found in the blood that assist in clotting. Aspirin works by inhibiting the clumping tendency of platelets.

Polyunsaturated fat
A type of fat found in vegetable oils and margarines that does not appear to raise blood cholesterol levels.

Post-pericardiotomy syndrome: Dressler's Syndrome
A build up of excess fluid between the heart and the membrane that surrounds it, often due to inflammation after open heart surgery.

Premature atrial contraction (PAC)
An early heartbeat that starts in the atria.

Premature ventricular contraction (PVC)
An early heartbeat that starts in the ventricles.

Prophylaxis
Prevention. Often refers to taking antibiotics prior to dental work to prevent heart valve infections.

Pulmonary
Pertaining to the respiratory system and lungs.

Pulmonary artery
The blood vessel connecting the right ventricle to the lungs, allowing oxygen-poor blood to receive oxygen.

Pulmonary edema
A severe form of congestive heart failure in which there is fluid accumulation in the lungs caused by an incorrectly functioning heart.

Pulmonary valve
The heart valve located between the right ventricle and the pulmonary artery that controls blood flow to the lungs.

Pulmonary vein
The vessel that carries oxygenated blood from the lungs to the left side of the heart.

Pulse oximeter
A device that measures the amount of oxygen in the blood. Normal oxygen saturation in the arteries is 95 to 100 percent.

Radioisotope
A radioactive material injected into the body so that a nuclear scanner can make pictures.

Regurgitation
Backward flow of blood caused by a defective heart valve.

Renal
Pertaining to the kidneys.

Rheumatic fever
A disease caused by a strep infection that may damage the heart valves.

Right atrium
The upper right chamber of the heart, which receives oxygen-poor (blue) blood from the body and sends it to the right ventricle.

Right ventricle
The lower right chamber of the heart, which receives oxygen-poor (blue) blood from the right atrium and sends it to the pulmonary artery.

Risk factor
A condition, element, or activity that may adversely affect the heart.

Ross procedure
A surgical procedure performed to repair aortic stenosis. The patient's own pulmonary valve and base of the pulmonary artery (autograft) replace the defective aorta, while a homograft (blood

vessel from a tissue donor) replaces the pulmonary valve and base of the pulmonary artery.

Saturated fat
Fat that is found in foods from animal meats and skin, dairy products, and some vegetables. Saturated fats are usually solid at room temperature and can increase LDL levels.

Septal defect
A hole in the wall between the atria or the ventricles (upper or lower heart chambers).

Septum
The muscle wall between the atria or ventricles (upper or lower heart chambers). The septum separates the right heart chambers from the left heart chambers.

Shunt
A connector to allow blood flow between two locations.

Sinus node
The cells that produce the electrical impulses that cause the heart to contract.

Sinus rhythm
A normal heart rhythm in which each heartbeat originates in the sinus node, and proceeds through the rest of the electrical conduction system normally.

Sinus tachycardia
A heart rhythm that originates in the sinus node and proceeds through the rest of the electrical conduction system, but is faster than normal.

Sphygmomanometer
An instrument used to measure blood pressure.

Stent
A small metal tube that is implanted in a narrowed blood vessel to keep it open.

Stenosis
Narrowing or constriction of a blood vessel or valve in the heart.

Stethoscope
An instrument used to listen to the heart and other sounds in the body.

Sternotomy
A surgical incision made in the breastbone.
Sternum
The breastbone.
Stroke
The sudden disruption of blood flow to the brain, often causes weakness on one side of the body or slurred speech.
Subclavian
A blood vessel that branches from the aorta and takes oxygen-rich (red) blood to the head and arms. It runs under the skin along the collar bone.
Superior vena cava
The large vein that returns blood to the heart from the head and arms.
Supraventricular tachycardia
A fast heart rate that originates in the aorta, but does not start in the sinus node.
Syncope
Light-headedness or fainting caused by insufficient blood supply to the brain.
Systole
The time during the heartbeat when the ventricles are pumping blood, either to the lungs or to the body.
Systolic blood pressure
The highest blood pressure measured in the arteries.
Tachycardia
Rapid heartbeat.
Tachypnea
Rapid breathing.
Tamponade
An emergency situation that occurs when blood or fluid fills the pericardial sac surrounding the heart, preventing the heart from beating effectively.
Thoracotomy
An incision made on the right or left side of the chest between the ribs, in order to access the heart or lungs during surgery.

TIA
Transient Ischemic Attack. A small stroke in which the symptoms resolve in 24 hours. Caused by tiny blood clots.

Trans fat
Vegetable oil that has been treated with hydrogen in order to make it more solid and give it a longer shelf life. Very harmful type of fat that contributes significantly to high cholesterol and is found in processed foods, cookies, crackers etc.

Transesophageal echocardiography (TEE)
A diagnostic test that uses a long tube guided into the mouth, throat, and esophagus to evaluate the structures inside the heart with sound waves. A much more detailed image of the heart is obtained than by the conventional echocardiogram.

Transplantation
Replacing a damaged organ with one from a donor.

Tricuspid valve
The heart valve that controls blood flow from the right atrium into the right ventricle.

Triglyceride
A fat-like substance found in the blood. A contributing factor to heart disease, more so in women than in men.

Ultrasound
A diagnostic tool used to evaluate organs and structures inside the body with high-frequency sound waves.

Valves
The one-way "doors" between the chambers of the heart that allow blood to move forward and prevent it from moving backward. The heart valves are called tricuspid, pulmonic, mitral, and aortic.

Valvuloplasty
Repairing a heart valve (as opposed to replacing it).

Vascular
Pertaining to blood vessels.

Vasodilator
A medication that dilates or widens the opening in a blood vessel.

Vasovagal syndrome
A sudden drop in blood pressure, with or without a decrease in heart rate, that is caused by a dysfunction of the nerves controlling the heart and blood vessels. The response is often precipitated by pain or fear.

Vein
A blood vessel that carries "old," deoxygenated blood from the body back into the heart to receive oxygen.

Ventricle
One of the two lower chambers of the heart.

VEGF
Vascular Endothelial Growth Factor. A substance produced by genes that stimulates growth of new blood vessels. ECP treatment stimulates the release of VEGF.

Ventricular fibrillation
A condition in which the ventricles contract in rapid and unsynchronized rhythms and cannot pump blood into the body. Unless immediately corrected, leads to sudden death.

Ventricular septal defect
An abnormal opening in the wall between the right and left ventricles.

Ventricular tachycardia
A condition in which the ventricles beat very quickly and may lead to sudden death.

Vertigo
Dizziness, usually described as a spinning sensation. Originates from malfunction of the balancing system of the middle ear.

Wolff-Parkinson-White syndrome
An extra electrical pathway that connects the atria and ventricles and causes rapid heartbeat.

About The Authors

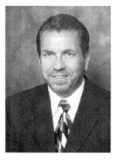

Dr. Lawrence J. Santora, M.D.

Dr. Santora is in private cardiology practice at the *Orange County Heart Institute and Research Center* in Orange County, California.

Dr. Santora did his undergraduate training at the University of Miami, Florida, then went on to receive his medical degree from New York Medical College. His cardiology training and Cardiology Fellowship were completed at the University of California at Irvine.

In the area of research, Dr. Santora was involved in studying the effects of liquid protein diets on cardiac function and heart rhythms in obese patients. His recent research involved ECP (external counterpulsation, a non-invasive treatment for angina) in the treatment of congestive heart failure. The study demonstrated significant benefits. He is the Director of Cardiac CT at The Orange County Heart Institute and OC Vital Imaging. His recently published research involved using EBCT heart scans to evaluate the effects of steroid use in elite bodybuilders. This is the first study ever to show a relationship between steroid abuse and heart disease. An alarmingly high degree of hardening of the coronary arteries in steroid users was noted, at a relatively young age.

Dr. Santora's clinical practice involves interventional cardiology, as well as preventive cardiology. He has partnered with Dick Butkus, of NFL Hall of Fame, and the Taylor Hooten Foundation to bring awareness of the dangers of steroid abuse in high school sports.

Dr. Santora recently co-authored, with Dick Butkus and Dr. Armentrout, *The OC Cure for Heart Disease.* This book describes an approach to heart disease using EBCT heart scans to detect coronary calcium, and a unique diet and exercise program. Also soon available, *A Cardiologist's Guide to Controlling High Blood Pressure,* by Dr. Azer and Dr. Santora. The **ocheart.org** Web site will announce the release of this book.

If you wish to order *Women and Heart Disease* on line, go to the following Web address: www.ocheart.org

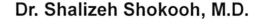

Dr. Shalizeh Shokooh, M.D.

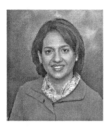

Dr. Shokooh is a Board Certified Cardiologist in private practice at the *Orange County Heart Institute and Research Center* in Orange County, California.

Dr. Shokooh completed her undergraduate studies at University of California, Irvine, where she also received her medical degree. She then completed her Internal Medicine training at University of California, San Diego, and University of California, Irvine. Her Cardiology training was at Harbor-UCLA Medical Center in California. During her training, she lectured on women and heart disease to nursing programs and was involved in EBCT research. Her research paper was published in 2002. She is currently the co-medical director at the St. Joseph Women's Heart Center in Orange, California. Her leadership at the center and her interest in preventing heart disease in women has been the driving force in her involvement in increasing awareness in the community. For the past three years she has been on the Board of Directors of the Orange County American Heart Association chapter. She has been actively involved in the *Go Red for Women* campaign and received the AHA Outstanding Medical Honoree award in February 2007. Her practice is focused on invasive and preventive cardiology with emphasis on women and heart disease.

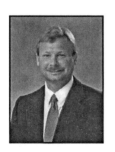

Dr. Kelly Tucker, M.D.

Dr. Tucker received his medical degree from the Uniformed Services University in Bethesda, Maryland. After serving in the United States Navy, Dr. Tucker completed fellowship training in Cardiac Imaging, Cardiovascular Diseases, and Cardiac Electrophysiology at the University of California, San Francisco, and University of Florida, Gainesville. Currently, Dr. Tucker is the director of Cardiac Electrophysiology and Pacing at the Orange County Heart Institute and an internationally renowned expert in cardiac arrhythmia management.

Index

Index

E

F

G

H

P

R

Printed in the United States
126950LV00003B/217-321/P

9 781886 571259